UNDERSTANDING

MENOPAUSE

UNDERSTANDING MENOPAUSE

JANINE O'LEARY COBB

KEY PORTER BOOKS

National Library of Canada Cataloguing in Publication Data

Cobb, Janine O'Leary, 1933–
 Understanding menopause

Rev. ed.
Includes bibliographical references and index.
ISBN 1-55263-375-6

1. Menopause. I. Title.

RG186.C62 2001   618.1'75   C2001-901433-3

THE CANADA COUNCIL | LE CONSEIL DES ARTS
FOR THE ARTS | DU CANADA
SINCE 1957 | DEPUIS 1957

The publisher gratefully acknowledges the support of the Canada Council for the
Arts and the Ontario Arts Council for its publishing program.

We acknowledge the financial support of the Government of Canada through the
Book Publishing Industry Development Program (BPIDP) for our publishing activities.

Key Porter Books Limited
70 The Esplanade
Toronto, Ontario
Canada M5E 1R2

www.keyporter.com

Publisher's Note: The contents of this book are not intended to be used as a
substitution for consultation with your physician. All matters pertaining to your
health should be directed to a health care professional.

Printed and bound in Canada

01 02 03 04 05 6 5 4 3 2 1

Certainly the effort to remain unchanged, young,
when the body gives so impressive a signal of change
as the menopause, is gallant; but it is a stupid,
self-sacrificial gallantry better befitting a boy of twenty
than a woman of forty-five or fifty.

Ursula K. Le Guin, "The Space Crone"

CONTENTS

INTRODUCTION
TO THE REVISED
EDITION

It has been 13 years since this book first appeared and I feel gratified when I still come across it on bookstore shelves. I'm gratified that I'm still around, too – well past my menopausal years but feeling fit as a fiddle.

Three years ago, I abandoned the day-to-day concerns of my newsletter, *A Friend Indeed*, to the tender ministrations of the Women's Health Clinic in Winnipeg, Manitoba, and a competent editor, Sari Tudiver. After a period of acting as official consultant, I can now relax and enjoy the arrival of the newsletter in the mail – just as many of you do six times a year.

This is a great change from the days when I spent all day, every day, studying and writing about menopause. Once I had a library of a few hundred books, all devoted to menopause, sitting on the shelf behind me. Those books are now part of the Women's Studies Library at the University of Toronto. Most were listed in the Bibliography which formed part of earlier editions of this book. Alas, most of these books are now out of print so listing them would be a potential exercise in frustration for my readers.

As I write this, Indigo Books and Chapters are still in the process of merging so I can't tell you where to order additional books on menopause. All I know is that the current <chapters.ca> has 195 books with "menopause" in the title, while <amazon.com> lists 173.

I am familiar with all the books prior to 1998 but I can't recommend any of the more recent ones.

I have some mementos of the days I spent focusing on menopause issues: a plaque from the North American Menopause Society "in appreciation of [my] contribution to the Education Committee, 1996, 1997" and a crystal flame in recognition of "Educational Excellence, 1998." The money accompanying that award enabled me to buy the laptop that I'm typing on right now.

Since I am no longer involved with the researchers and physicians who generate information about menopause, I can be more candid about what I saw and heard over the fourteen years that I worked exclusively on one topic. In the early years (1984–1990), when I attended meetings of the International Menopause Society and the nascent North American Menopause Society, I was thoroughly shocked at the quality of many of the medical reports. These were studies based on twelve or fourteen or eighteen women, each of whom was a patient (hardly representative of healthy menopausal women), and each of whom had come to that doctor with some sort of problem. I didn't consider myself a research scientist, but I was aghast that these small numbers of atypical women should lead doctors to conclusions that were too often presented as applying to menopausal women generally.

As menopause generated more interest, the quality of the research improved. But it was instructive to realize that so many of the early studies of menopause were based on such fragile premises. (One of the best-known "names" in the area of sexuality during menopause continued to produce such questionable reports for years.)

Later, as I became more immersed in menopause research, I began to know the names and recognize the faces of these well-known menopause doctors. What I perceived was a yawning chasm between physician/clinicians, who were on the front lines, seeing women beaten up by menopause, and physician/researchers. The researchers almost inevitably considered themselves superior to the clinicians, but it was the clinicians who were more cognizant of the manifold factors impinging on a woman's health in midlife – pressures of work, from husbands, from children, from parents.

On the other hand, the clinicians were – and are – often too busy to read the latest research. Instead, they tend to rely on reprints of research articles brought to them by the "detail men" – the pharmaceutical representatives who drop in from time to time. These are often studies published in prestigious journals like the *New England Journal of Medicine*, the *Journal of the American Medical Association* (*JAMA*), *Obstetrics & Gynecology*, or *Lancet* (the premier British medical journal) so they command a certain amount of respect.

But they are nearly always articles chosen to favor the representative's company's products and, as I have discovered, many of the research topics are proposed to the researchers by the pharmaceutical company's research department. The pharmaceutical company then pays for the product, the placebo, and sometimes the cost of doing the research. Sometimes they even provide a ghost writer. Even when the publication requires researchers to reveal affiliations with or funding from pharmaceutical companies – and this is not always the case – the conflict of interest appears in small print at the end of the article.

The ideal of science is to generate objective facts. As I have realized – to my dismay – that process is too often cluttered by vested interests that guide the results to a desired conclusion.

What I have tried to do in this book is supply citations from the medical literature to back up any assertions that I make that may be contrary to what your doctor tells you. These references appear at the back of the book, and I urge you to look at them when and if I make statements that you or your doctor find hard to believe. The titles of the articles will guide you. If you need a copy of the article cited, this can be obtained at any medical library. Often, the abstracts (a summary of the relevant findings) can be downloaded from the internet.

Now that I'm retired, I am not just sitting idly twiddling my thumbs. Since my own mercifully brief encounter with breast cancer in 1998, I have become involved on a voluntary basis with Breast Cancer Action Montreal, an organization that struggles to increase awareness of the causes and prevention of breast cancer. And it *is* a struggle, when most of the mainstream breast cancer organizations have chosen to devote their time, and 97 percent of their dollars, to research into screening and treatment.

I'm also involved with a coalition of American and Canadian women's health organizations that are battling against the insidious promotion of prescription medications to the general public. This is supposed to be banned in Canada but we are exposed to great amounts of overflow advertising from the States, and the U.S. Food & Drug Administration admits that they don't have the manpower to supervise it.

We are also traveling when we can find the time and the money. We really enjoy it. And then, just before I started to write this introduction, we were told that our tenth grandchild is on its way. My days are full, my gratitude is boundless.

– April 2001

INTRODUCTION
TO THE FIRST
EDITION

It was my intention that my forty-ninth summer be memorable. I planned to spend most of that summer in the country, taking possession of the cottage that we had dreamed about for years. I also planned to give up smoking – this time for good – as a fiftieth-birthday present to myself, and to write a text for a course I had been developing, to be taught as part of the humanities program at Vanier College in Montreal. I had been smoking steadily and heavily for almost thirty years; I needed a peaceful and ordered existence if I was to stop smoking and write a book. Fortunately, four of my five children were working or were at camp; the youngest would be pleasant company during the week, and my husband would arrive on Friday afternoons for the weekend.

The cottage got built, the manuscript was finished, and I haven't smoked since, but that summer is memorable for other reasons. Looking back, I remember the sudden fits of warmth during the night (except for pregnancy, I had never been *too* warm!), the aching right shoulder (which forced me to swim sidestroke, when I preferred the Australian crawl), and the weird dreams of giving birth or of waking to a bed flooded with menstrual fluid. I didn't realize it at the time, but the summer constituted a turning point – an unconscious farewell to the closure of my reproductive life.

Over the following academic year, I continued to teach my sociology and humanities classes. The usual routine of preparation, classes, and marking was overshadowed by threatened changes to the college system – changes that would drastically increase the numbers of students in the classroom and, at the same time, shrink the amount of time available for classroom preparation and grading. I was also coping with a full house: my two elder sons had been away from home and had returned to go back to school. I thought I would never live through Christmas, with all its attendant responsibilities. By the time classes got under way in January, I was in the throes of a full-fledged depression.

Because I was still menstruating, I never seriously thought of menopause. I believed (from what little I knew) that menopause was a problem only to women who had time on their hands. As a full-time college professor, wife, and mother, I had no time for menopausal distress. When I complained about my lagging capacity for coping, I discovered that most of my same-age friends were feeling similarly. Some were having serious problems with children; some were making noises about leaving their husbands; all were talking about "burnout" and the inability to feel enthusiastic about their jobs. And *none* of us attributed any of this to menopause.

I celebrated my fiftieth birthday in the south of France – my first trip to Europe and a glorious birthday present from a husband who was, by this time, turning cartwheels in an effort to cheer me up. I continued to feel grim, weepy, and pessimistic about everything, but I wouldn't see a doctor, because I was convinced I had no *reason* to feel depressed. I refused to discuss the matter and I grew accustomed to the strange glances from family members.

By Christmas of that year (the year we bought a computer as a gift for the children), I had done a bit of research on menopause. I had browsed through the Health section of the bookstores, looking for a paragraph, a chapter, something that would give me a clue. I had found some interesting material (for example, Rosetta Reitz's book, *Menopause: A Positive Approach*, and a chapter in Penny Wise Budoff's first book, *No More Menstrual Cramps and Other Good News*), but I was beginning to get angry about the general lack of information. At my annual checkup, the doctor had mentioned a discussion group on menopause, adding that it was primarily informational (information that I had already found for myself), but that it might provide moral support. I didn't have time to register or to attend – I was about to start a course in word processing. As I became familiar with the capabilities of the computer, it all started to come together.

I got the idea for a newsletter for menopausal women that could be both a source of information and a support group *through the mail*. In March 1984, I carefully printed out a trial newsletter and mailed it to any and every woman I had ever met or heard about who might be interested. Because menopause is a time when a woman often *is* in need, I called it *A Friend Indeed*.

Since that first tentative mailing to forty women, *A Friend Indeed* has grown steadily. During the first summer, a newspaper article was reprinted across the country: a week later, I had received more than nine hundred inquiries. After the next Christmas, I taught only half-time and introduced a French version, *Une véritable amie*. By September 1985, I was working full-time on the newsletter, as I continue to do now.

The success of *A Friend Indeed* is due, in large measure, to the caring and sharing of thousands of menopausal women across Canada. Through their letters, some of which are reproduced in the chapters of this book, I have learned to esteem highly the knowledge and judgment of women "in the prime of life." Although the decision to invest all my energy in the newsletter has meant unaccustomed isolation (me and my computer) and, at times, downright loneliness, when I do emerge from my office to travel to other cities or to attend a conference or workshop, I am warmed by the spontaneous kindnesses and friendly hospitality I receive.

Although I had thought that the newsletter would suffice, readers have persuaded me that a compendium, complete with index and "ready reference," might be even more useful and might, in fact, be appealing to many women who are not yet ready to accept the adjective "menopausal." This book is for the women in their early forties who are, perhaps unknowingly, dealing with the minor changes that precede menopause: it is my hope that the information you find will alleviate any irrational apprehension. This book is also for those passing through menopause. Understanding what is happening will, I think, allow you to reestablish cordial relations with a body and mind that might be temporarily out of whack, thus enabling you to manage your menopause with confidence.

I am grateful to my family, who have put up with, and come to the aid of, a wife/mother who takes on too much, and is often too intense, too earnest, and too easily upset. I love each of you more than I can say. I am grateful above all to the women who have become my subscribers and my friends, and to the women who were always my friends and have now become my subscribers. You have opened my eyes to new ways of seeing this transitional period in our lives. Let me say it: menopause has been a very *special* time.

– June 1988

CHAPTER 1

HOW TO RECOGNIZE THE ONSET OF MENOPAUSE

Once upon a time, women were deliberately kept in ignorance of the measured steps of womanhood and the role of their own reproductive organs in menstruation, sexual intercourse, pregnancy, and menopause. Each event arrived unheralded and unknown. Today most females in this society are encouraged to know something about each, but the least known of them all is menopause.

During the past two or three decades, women have become conscious of entrenched sexist attitudes toward many solely female experiences – menstruation, pregnancy, childbirth. These important events in a woman's life have never been taken too seriously by the male political or medical establishments. These attitudes are changing, thanks in large part to the activism of younger women. Midlife women may not be as assertive. Many are faced with not only sexist attitudes, but also ageist attitudes that discount and dismiss the very real concerns of menopausal women. Rather than label ourselves as "menopausal" and thereby invite the negative stereotype of the middle-aged complainer, too many of us keep silent. Sadly, ignorance of our bodily processes feeds fear.

Isn't it strange that we should be educated in the intricacies of sexual intercourse, pregnancy, and childbirth – which are never experienced by *all women* – yet left virtually uneducated about a process that touches *each one*? All we have to do is live long enough. These days, most women do.

> I didn't recognize the first signs of menopause. I assumed, since I was working full-time outside the home and leading a full and satisfying life, that I would be relatively untouched by it. When I finally saw a doctor about my sore wrists, I was told that it often happened "for no reason" and that there was no reliable cure. When I started feeling depressed, I assumed it was because of the constant insecurity and stress experienced by any woman in my kind of job. It got a lot worse before I belatedly recognized that menopause might be responsible.

For most of our adult lives, we are governed by cycles that are more or less predictable. Even those of us who menstruate rarely are accustomed to a predictable unpredictability of menses, or periods. The vast majority become accustomed to menstrual cycles that fall within a given time frame – always early when you don't want the bother; always late when you count on getting it over with by a certain date! By the age of twenty, most of us have learned to gauge the numbers of tampons and/or pads required and to schedule our lives around the inevitable arrival of "that time of the month." We may have even learned to laugh (in retrospect) at our excessive emotionality during the days just before menstruation. Many of us have also learned to get back into the swing after months of pregnancy and/or breast feeding. The menstrual cycle is a familiar rhythm, and although we complain that it's inconvenient (or worse), we have grown accustomed to it.

This familiarity with one's menstrual cycle is very difficult for a man to understand. Because women complain about the way menstrual cycles govern their lives, men think that we hate menstruation and want to be rid of it. Some women do. But most learn to accommodate the vagaries of menstruation and to make allowances for it. As with an unruly pet, you complain about it, but you can't imagine doing without it.

There is considerable time devoted to the accommodation of menstruation – and the time of adaptation begins even *before* menarche (the first menstrual period), when a girl's body is readying itself to menstruate. The cycle gradually regulates itself; once it is established, there follows the adjustment to the physical and emotional ups and downs that occur every month. A girl who starts menstruating at about age thirteen will probably take at least five years to adjust to, and be comfortable with, her cycle and its intricate effects – emotional, psychological, and physical. Those of us who think back to our adolescence should not be surprised if, after thirty-five years, we require five years or more to readapt to *not* menstruating.

This is menopause.

If you look up the word *menopause* in a dictionary, you will not find "a five- to seven-year period marking the end of the reproductive years in women." What you *will* find is "the cessation of menstruation" – a point in time that comes and goes before most of us notice.

There are some problems with this definition. First of all, naturally menopausal women can only acknowledge menopause in retrospect. We never know which menstrual period is the last until it is over. Second, there are many women who experience a last menstrual period as the result of surgical (or other artificial) interventions but who are not necessarily menopausal. An alternative, more correct, term is *climacteric*, which comes from a Greek term suggesting steps on a ladder and which covers the whole midlife period for both males and females. Changes were thought to take place every seven years, and the odd multiples, such as thirty-five, forty-nine, and sixty-three, were considered very important.

Ancient Greek society revolved around the needs and perceptions of men, but because this is a book written *by* a woman and largely *for* women, I'm going to use *menopause* in its commonly accepted sense: as a transitional period marking the closure of reproductive life, usually but not always occurring during midlife. *Menopause* in this book refers, according to common usage, to a "time of life" rather than a "point in time."

The average age at which a woman in North America has her

last menstrual period is fifty-one, but it may come earlier in some families and later in others. Any time between forty and fifty-nine falls within the realm of "normal." Age at first menstruation seems to have little to do with the start of menopause. Length of cycle and numbers of pregnancies may have some bearing; women who cycle every twenty-six days or so will have an earlier menopause than women who cycle every thirty-three days. Smoking will bring on an earlier menopause (up to two years earlier for a heavy smoker), and a hysterectomy (removal of the uterus) and/or tubal ligation (tying or cauterization of the fallopian tubes to ensure infertility) lead to earlier menopause *in some cases*. This may be contrary to what you have been told by your doctor. The findings I cite (Cattanach, 1985) are from an old study and based on small numbers. Although there has been an unfortunate lack of interest in replicating this study, when coupled with anecdotal evidence, I suspect it may well hold.

Natural Menopause

A disturbance in the monthly cycle may or may not be the first sign of onset of menopause. Throughout most of our adult lives, the menstrual cycle operates in a more-or-less expected way, with hormones ebbing and flowing at levels just high enough to keep the system in comfortable balance. As you get closer to the last menstrual period, fluctuations occur – fluctuations that may affect menstruation so little as not to be noticed but that may give you something to wonder about. Many women notice changes in bowel habits or stools; others notice headaches that come and go more frequently. There may be a difference in energy levels or the content of dreams. Many women find that their joints – knees or ankles, wrists or shoulders – start to ache for no reason. Some women experience increased premenstrual distress (PMS). Others report many, very *minor* complaints at their regular checkups. Yet, paradoxically, life may be treating them well in most other ways: Many women are financially more stable than in their twenties; have had time to experience the satisfactions of accomplishment, personally or professionally; and have come to terms with their physical appearance. It is only hindsight that enables many of us to recognize slight changes that occur during the early forties, changes that precede the better-known signs of menopause.

The Normal Reproductive Cycle

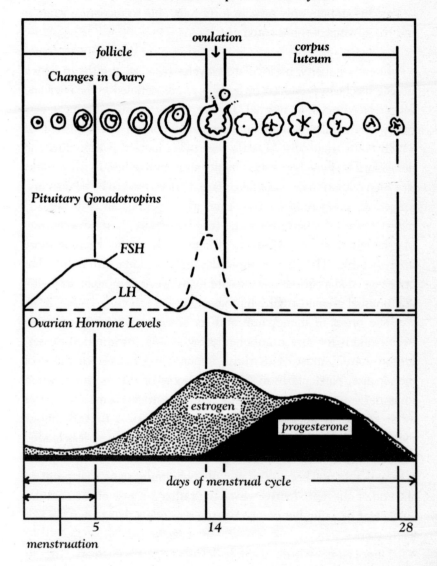

A few years ago, I went to see my doctor regarding a pounding in my heart and aches in my joints. He never even suggested it might be menopause, stating that, at forty-two, I was too young. Thinking back, I believe it started when I was thirty-nine or forty years old. I experienced minor symptoms as early as this and am only now, at forty-four, able to recognize what these symptoms indicated.

In early puberty, nonovulatory cycles (that is, months in which no egg has been produced by an ovary) are signaled by heavier and longer bleeding than normal. In fact, many young girls have very heavy or irregular periods *until* regular ovulation is established, at which point their periods settle down to a more tolerable flow and duration. The same happens as menopause approaches. In the months in which ovulation does *not* take place, periods tend to be heavier and longer. As premenopause (the time when periods are still regular) moves toward the perimenopause (the transition phase between regular periods and no periods at all), monthly events become more unpredictable. The two or three days of emotional instability that once preceded a period may escalate into a week or more of annoying and unusual premenstrual symptoms.

The onset of menopause and its accompanying ailments can be mistaken for any number of slow-acting, terminal illnesses. Unfortunately, most of us think about dying before we think of menopause, particularly in the small hours of the morning, when imaginations run rampant. This tendency to view menopause as a "sickness" is accentuated by our inclination to talk about menopause *symptoms*. In this book, I have tried to use less loaded terms – "signs," "indications," "ailments." The onset of menopause is remarkable not because of any overwhelming signs that point to the end of our reproductive years, but rather because of the cumulative effect of a number of aggravating reminders that things are not as they once were.

Menopause, by itself, is rarely devastating. It is estimated that in this society only a small minority (10 to 15 percent) of naturally menopausal women will experience severe or debilitating symptoms. Another small minority (perhaps 10 percent) will sail through with no problems whatsoever. This leaves the rest of us somewhere in the middle. Some have a rocky time but cope without drugs or other medical interventions. Others experience only infrequent and mild reminders of their menopausal status. It is the sensation of a loss of control over one's own body that is often the worst problem. If you have a reasonable idea of what to expect, managing the situation is much easier.

Artificial Menopause

There can be a significant difference between the menopause experience of a woman who has had her uterus removed (that is, who has had a hysterectomy) and a woman whose organs are intact. A substantial number of women who have had hysterectomies, *whether or not any part of the ovaries has been saved,* experience either premature menopause or a menopause quite different from that of a naturally menopausal woman. Women who have both ovaries removed (an oophorectomy, or ovariectomy), or whose ovaries fail as a result of chemotherapy, will have a different kind of menopause; women who have other kinds of medical interventions (tubal ligation, complete or partial hysterectomy, radiation treatment, etc.), may not be sure whether they will have a completely natural menopause, premature menopause, or artificial menopause. (Younger women often recover from chemotherapy to resume menstruating, but women in their forties seldom do.) Rarely do physicians give their patients a clear explanation of what to expect after such intervention.

Many women are unaware of the extent of their own surgery. A *complete hysterectomy*, in everyday language, usually means removal of the uterus, cervix, ovaries, and fallopian tubes. But to a doctor, a complete hysterectomy means removal of the uterus and cervix only. It is important for a woman to know exactly what organs are involved in surgery if she is to understand the reasons for, and the possible consequences of, the operation.

For instance, until fairly recently, it was thought that the experience of menopause was similar for any woman who still had her ovaries or part of them – that even a small part of one ovary would continue to secrete enough estrogen to allow for menopause at the normal age. We now know that is not true, that in many cases the remaining ovarian tissue simply cannot continue to function adequately.

The term *artificial menopause* may be applied to: (1) those women who have had their ovaries removed (usually in conjunction with a hysterectomy); (2) those whose ovaries fail following radiation or chemotherapy; (3) those who experience a premature menopause as a result of a hysterectomy, even when some or all of the ovaries are untouched.

The women in categories (1) and (2) experience a very sudden menopause. The hot flashes start within a few days of surgery (or treatment) and may be brutal in their effects. At the same time, a number of other ailments may strike all at once – headaches, joint pains, fatigue, night sweats, depression, etc. Unless there are good reasons to avoid it, estrogen therapy (ET)* is started almost immediately and may continue for some years.

The risk of depression is high for women in all three categories, with the incidence highest about two years after hysterectomy. In addition, women whose ovaries cease functioning before age forty will be at increased risk for both osteoporosis and heart disease. This is why all young women should work hard to develop bone mass, through diet and exercise, and why the experiences of natural menopause and artificial menopause should be considered separately.

Women who retain all or some of their ovaries are less severely

---

* In cases where the ovaries have been removed or rendered inoperative, estrogen therapy is administered as estrogen replacement therapy (ERT). This is how any form of estrogen therapy appears in most of the literature on menopause. But ERT only "replaces" lost estrogen when it is given to women who experience an abnormal depletion of estrogen, either as a result of medical intervention or because of premature ovarian failure. Estrogen administered to women who go through natural menopause at the expected age replaces nothing, since it is perfectly normal for estrogen to be reduced at this time of life. Therefore, estrogen therapy is referred to as ET throughout this book. Similarly, hormone therapy using estrogen and progestins (synthetic progesterone) is referred to as combined hormone therapy (CHT).

affected. However, in from one-third to one-half of cases, menopause may occur prematurely. The closer one is to age fifty at the time of the surgery, the more likely it is that menopause will be advanced; according to studies, women who are hysterectomized before the age of forty will experience menopause an average of eight years after surgery.

> After undergoing a hysterectomy at age twenty-seven, I believe I am now experiencing menopause. I am forty-one years old. The symptoms started about four years ago and have included tingling sensations, anxiety, hot flashes, severe panic attacks, and depression. Lately I've been feeling so poorly that I wish I could go to sleep and never wake up. The three doctors I've seen tell me I'm too young to be experiencing menopause.

Whether we experience natural or artificial menopause, we need information beforehand, and during the period of adjustment most of us can use some understanding and support. To receive understanding and support, we have to be both willing to admit our frailties and prepared to listen to and affirm the experiences of other women. Unfortunately, many women decide to unburden themselves only to one other woman. What if (as it may turn out) this person is one of the small minority who just stopped menstruating without any problem? Such women often take personal credit for a problem-free menopause (by "keeping busy," "not dwelling on things," or "having a sense of humor"). This is not very supportive of the woman suffering from menopausal distress! It is then that we start asking questions: Why am I saddled with all these problems, while she gets off painlessly? Is it heredity? Is it diet? Is it the cumulative effect of medication taken over the years? Is it the operation?

There are no real answers to these kinds of questions. Sisters usually have a similar experience of menopause and go through it at roughly the same age. When there are sharp differences, it forces us to question differences in diet, exercise, sleep habits, or previous hormone use – for adolescent acne, to induce ovulation, to prevent pregnancy, to induce delivery, to prevent miscarriage, to dry up breast milk, to alleviate hot flashes. The medical world knows very little about the effects of cumulative doses of hormones and how they might influence the age at which a woman goes through menopause, or the quality of the menopause itself.

Menopause and Aging

How much of a woman's experience is menopause and how much is aging? This is the million-dollar question. Because menopause and the sensation of aging often appear hand in hand, the careful separation of one from the other has become a matter of serious academic interest. Apparently, very few of the negatives can be directly attributed to menopause; depression, fatigue, anxiety, wrinkles, and gray hair are more easily linked to factors *other* than menopause. Many of the symptoms of premenstrual syndrome (PMS) – a few days of severe physical and emotional distress prior to the menstrual period – may be triggered by menopause (natural or surgical) and may continue to be felt on a regular cycle for months or years after the last menstrual period. If this is true, it means that chemicals in the brain produce many so-called menopausal ailments.

On the other hand, many of us know that we *have* visibly aged since our menstrual periods started to falter. Those of us who go gray in our late forties and early fifties, who find ourselves stuck with a substantial weight gain, and who also battle fatigue and aching joints, feel – not surprisingly – that menopause is responsible. In reality, it is very hard to separate aging from menopause.

It is not necessary to gain weight (although weight gain may have very positive benefits). The onset of menopause is a signal to start watching what you eat. If you feel unexpectedly tired at the end of a normal day, you would be wise to protect yourself from fatigue by cutting down on your commitments – to work, to family, to friends. Aches in joints will probably disappear in time. The good news is that the menopause doldrums will pass. Once your body has adjusted to your new nonmenstruating self, you will reach a more stable and pleasant stage of development – the plateau called postmenopause.

Postmenopause is established after you have been through twelve months without a menstrual period. Margaret Mead, the famous anthropologist, introduced the term *postmenopausal zest* to describe the feelings of renewed energy and health that mark women in this stage, women from their mid- to late-fifties onward. This is where one sees a sharp contrast between the listless newly retired man and his peppy, busy wife! The years after menopause are usually enormously productive.

Social Definitions of Menopause

The view of menopause differs widely from society to society. In some societies, the onset of menopause is welcomed because it provides a break from stringent rules about what women may or may not do or say. In other societies it is regarded as an inevitable part of growing older and viewed neither positively nor negatively. In our society, which makes a fetish of both youth and slimness, menopause is often dreaded. Many of us find, much to our dismay, that we have unconsciously subscribed to our society's very narrow definition of "femininity" and that we are not willing to look our age. To deal with this, it helps to examine the social standards for men, who are often seen as *more* attractive as they age. Gray-haired and portly, they project an air of self-confidence and prosperity and a well-weathered masculinity. This hard-earned confidence should also be incorporated into women's views of themselves at midlife, but it often takes a conscious effort to ignore, or to see beyond, the stereotype of the menopausal woman and to focus on the positive aspects of the menopausal years.

Such effort is required because there is, in our society, a sense of loss associated with menopause. It is not that we mourn the loss of the ability to have a baby. Most women are not interested in being new mothers at age fifty. Nor do we mourn the diminishing maternal role. Most of us are delighted to see our children step out on their own. What women mourn is the loss of their youthful image, which must now be replaced with a more mature, capable image.

The mantle of middle age descends with a thud. As Germaine Greer says:

> It isn't a gradual, imperceptible process, but happens in leaps and bounds. You can go on for years being the same age. Your face doesn't change much; your weight remains much the same. You never think of yourself as too old to learn the latest craze, can't wait to [get] off with the old and [get] on with the new. Then, crunch. You're polishing a mirror table and you realize your neck has gone. Just like that. ("Letting Go," *Vogue*, May 1986, p. 141)

If there were an expectation of new challenges and new adventures at age fifty, menopause would be looked at much more positively. Unfortunately, in this society, the expectations and markers are almost uniformly negative. Women approach menopause with attitudes that influence how they deal with it. Because we lack positive images of women coping with menopause, the attitudes tend to be negative.

> It just seems that menopause takes over one's whole life. I was a year getting over the feelings of I-really-don't-know-what. And all of a sudden I feel "old" and realize that life is now on the down half. Immediately one is no longer young and vital – just old and tired and useless.

And yet, if we keep our eyes open, we can see vital and healthy women in their fifties, sixties, seventies who have overcome this negativity. Look how far we've come in relation to the women of fifty or one hundred years ago!

Confronting Menopause

Some women choose to deny the existence of menopause. This is fairly easy in our society and reflects the common attitude of dread.

Unless there are definite medical reasons for not doing so, many doctors willingly prescribe hormones so that the monthly menstrual period will continue for some years. However, this means turning a blind eye to possible side effects and long-term consequences – in effect, abdicating responsibility for an informed choice. Women who choose to deal with menopause by avoiding it entirely are not hard to spot. Strenuous dieting, consistent application of hair color, and skillful application of makeup may minimize the effects of aging, but how long can they avoid it? What happens when time (and nature) catches up with them? How will they deal with a new "self" and an aging body – as someday we all must?

Some women give in to menopause and aging immediately. The first twinge of joint pain is interpreted as arthritis, and a sure sign of disability. Weight gain is viewed as both inevitable and an excuse for inactivity – particularly sexual activity. Anxiety and irritability are expected, often because a close friend or relative had problems at this age. With this kind of attitude, it is easy to sink into depression. As aches and pains multiply, visits to the doctor become more frequent. Because these women are the ones who turn up at doctors' offices, they too often come to personify the menopausal woman. These women are victims of our society's negative view of aging and illness, and these are the women who give menopause a bad name.

A few women will reach menopause and sail through with barely a twinge or a backward glance. We don't know why such women are spared, although – like the research on happy marriages – it would be nice to spread the good news. The vast majority of naturally menopausal women will be bothered to some extent by minor ailments that come and go over a period of years. With some basic information about diet, exercise, and nonprescription remedies, most women can live and cope very well. If they are also blessed with some sincere empathy and support from friends, most women can navigate the trickier stumbling blocks of menopause.

Regarding menopause, in all fairness to this process I must tell of spells of great well-being, which come rarely but are so strong and wonderful that I note them in my journal.

They last ten to fifteen minutes, and during that time I am totally content with the world. More than that, really. The sunshine and colors of my surroundings are perfect, my family is totally right and complete, my body and mind are just as they should be, and I am aware that all's right with the world. This is more difficult to put into words than I thought it would be. However, it is a marvelously aware and alive feeling and, I think, related to our time of life.

Yes, I have anxiety attacks and forgetfulness and mostly sleep loss, especially in the two weeks prior to my body's efforts to menstruate. My periods are getting lighter at last (I'll be fifty-three soon), but these "moments of perfection" are worth it.

The attitudes toward menopause and toward menopausal women in *this* society have been fabricated from false assumptions, rumor, fear of aging, and media hype. Recognizing the negativism of these attitudes helps me to understand why physicians are so insistent on "treating" us, why husbands want us to take pills so we will become the wives we used to be, why younger women are apprehensive about menopause, why middle-aged women are so frightened at the prospect of aging. At the same time, I think of other societies, past and present, where midlife women are held in esteem and given special status; where they are the repositories of wisdom and the counselors of their people. This could happen again.

My hope is that if each of us stresses the positive contributions made by the vibrant, capable midlife women in our midst (and that means you), we will change attitudes and make midlife and menopause stages of life to be anticipated – for our daughters and, even more, our granddaughters.

CHAPTER 2

PHYSICAL
AILMENTS
AT MENOPAUSE

Sometimes it's hard to believe that women have been going through menopause for centuries. We have very little information about what the experience was like for women before us, and until someone delves into the letters and diaries of our "foremothers," we have only the misleading accounts of the men who treated them. Because there *has* been so little information available about menopause, we tend to view it as an impediment that must be overcome so that we can get on with our lives. This, in turn has led to reassuring articles that tell us we will be past it in a few months or, at most, a couple of years. The purpose is to downplay the interruption and regard adult life as a continuous line. I believe this attitude does grave disservice to the experience of menopause and its effects.

Most other animals die as soon as their reproductive lives are over. The human female is the only one to survive for such a long time after the end of her reproductive life – an average of twenty-five to thirty years, or more than one-third of her lifespan. This uniquely human capacity is presumed to have evolved from the needs of the newborn human, who has an extraordinarily long dependency period, and ensures that "Mother" will be on hand for the needs of the last born. Even those who accept this as an evolutionary benefit, however, sometimes wonder why menopause operates in the way it does. Why does nature have to add so many hormonal upsets to the end of ovulation?

According to the theories of developmental psychology, everyone goes through stages of personality growth – periods of disruption followed by the incorporation of new learning and another step on the road to maturity. Each stage leads to new attitudes and behaviors that reflect the new learning. This is how we mature.

Most of us know something about the stages of childhood. We know that the path to maturity is marked with upheaval and that, all being well, the crises are followed by the emergence of a wiser, more self-sufficient child. The crises, of course, vary. It is hard sometimes to see the similarities among a two-year-old's tantrum, the stomach ache of a seven-year-old who doesn't want to go to school, and the heartbroken sobs of a lovestruck adolescent. But the downs of each of these episodes are usually followed by an up – a period of self-recognition and a new stage of self-knowledge on the way to adulthood.

When we look back on our adult lives, we can often pick out similar "growth spurts" – crises faced and dealt with and new insights gained as a result. At work, these steps can be fairly easily charted. Most of us can look back at a particular rocky period that marked the taking on of more responsibility or a new level of confidence about the job. We can also see that marriage, or the dissolution of marriage, requires nonstop accommodation to another personality, to another situation. Out of the pain comes growth and eventually stability, either with someone else or alone. Motherhood demands new skills every few years, skills that are not easy to learn. The best mothers of babies are not always the best mothers of adolescents (which is why many of us grow nostalgic about the simpler needs of very young children). To view our own adulthood as one unbroken line that moves onward into old age is to disregard the bumpy road that we have all traveled.

One of the myths of menopause is that one enters it, weathers it, and goes back to being the same woman, only older. This is to deny the essential truth of menopause: that it is a crucial stage of development on the road to maturity and that the experience will change us. Most women reach a new plateau of contentment *after* menopause.

✦

In order to understand what you are (or will be) experiencing during menopause, it is important to recognize a range of symptoms – both physical and psychological – that commonly affect women during this time. Although you almost certainly will not experience more than a few of these ailments, it helps to have heard about them just in case you *do* experience them.

Menopausal Ailments

menstrual irregularity
hot flashes and/or flushes; night sweats
dry vagina
insomnia and/or weird dreams
sensory disturbances (vision, smell, alterations to taste)
funny sensations in the head
lower back pain (crushing of vertebrae)
waking in the early hours of the morning
onset of new allergies or sensitivities
fluctuations in sexual desire and sexual response
annoying itching of the vulva (area around vagina)
sudden bouts of bloat (waistline expands by two to
    three inches for an hour or two)
chills or periods of extreme warmth
indigestion, flatulence (wind), gas pains
rogue chin whiskers
overnight appearance of long, fine facial hairs
bouts of rapid heartbeat
crying for no reason
aching ankles, knees, wrists, or shoulders
waking up with sore heels

thinning scalp and underarm hair
graying scalp and pubic hair
mysterious appearance of bruises
sudden inability to breathe ("air hunger")
frequent urination
urinary leakage (when coughing or sneezing,
    or during orgasm)
prickly or tingly hands with swollen veins
lightheadedness, dizzy spells, or vertigo
weight gain and in unusual places (on the back, breasts,
abdomen)
sudden and inappropriate bursts of anger
sensitivity to touching by others ("touch impairment")
inexplicable panic attacks
tendency to cystitis (inflammation of the bladder)
vaginal or urethral infections
anxiety and loss of self-confidence
depression that cannot be shaken off
painful intercourse
migraine headaches
easily wounded feelings
crawly skin ("formication")
disturbing memory lapses

Despite the documented occurrence of all the ailments listed, most medical texts recognize only three major physical ailments: menstrual irregularity, hot flashes, and dry vagina (or genitourinary distress). Osteoporosis is occasionally listed as a symptom of menopause, but it is, in fact, a condition that begins long before menopause and only sometimes becomes critical during the menopausal years. Psychological ailments (anxiety, panic attacks, and depression) are viewed in very different ways, depending on the source or the expert you consult. The three major physical ailments (sometimes expanded to four with the addition of osteoporosis) that follow are the ones that most doctors are prepared to discuss and treat.

Standard Signs Of Menopause

Menstrual irregularity

The most common sign of menopause is a fluctuation in the menstrual cycle. Although this may not be the *first* indication of menopausal onset, it is the one most women look for. Periods may continue to arrive on time, but there are often minor changes. The woman who once could relax for an hour or two between the "show" and the need for a pad or tampon may find that she is now quickly staining her clothes. The period that lasted three or four days may last for two or six. The color of the flow may change – rather than moving from red to brown, it may be brown, then red, then brown again. All this is normal, as is the increasing tendency to skip a period now and then, or to have two or three periods back to back. If you are familiar with your own rhythm, you will be more exasperated by all this than alarmed.

> The cessation of my menstrual periods was gradual. It lasted for approximately three years, and the uncertainty was most irritating and often quite embarrassing. I experienced minor symptoms of menopause, such as light-headedness and hot flashes, during this time. However, now that my periods have ceased altogether, menopause has arrived in full force. I am experiencing hot flashes, mood swings, and dry vagina. I realize now that it is specifically during the first signs of menopause – that is, erratic menses – that one should take the opportunity to inform oneself fully about the years to follow.

What is *not* normal is bleeding between periods. If you experience this, be sure to consult your doctor.

Hot flashes and night sweats

Another very common physical symptom is the hot flash. In North America, we say "flash"; in England, it is commonly "flush." But they are not necessarily the same thing. A hot flash is the sudden sensation of heat (it may be experienced as a result of stress in the absence of menopause). A hot flush is the red neck or face that is visible to others. (You may have a red chest or back as well.) You can have a flush without feeling a flash, and you can feel a flash without "giving it away" with a flush. Hot flashes experienced during the night are called night sweats. Some women experience flashes but no night sweats; some experience only night sweats; some experience both. And some women don't have hot flashes; they have cold chills, which is just a variation.

The onset of hot flashes is often heralded by the unexpected return of the old-fashioned "blush." Many women find their faces reddening without feeling any sensation of warmth. The first experience of a hot flash may be nothing more than a feeling of unusual warmth; you may throw the covers off or remove a jacket or sweater, and not think about it further. Doctors estimate that between 75 and 85 percent of North American women experience hot flashes, although general population surveys put the number at around 40 to 50 percent. Some women have hot flashes for only a few weeks and some for as long as fifteen to twenty years. Many women feel some sort of premonition before a hot flash starts. In studies done of hot flashes, women are often able to say, "Here comes one!" before the medical instruments start to show any differences in skin temperature or blood circulation. After the signal there is frequently a rapid build-up – often concentrated in the chest and upper body – in body temperature and a feeling of unbearable heat. The veins of the hands may tingle and swell. Perspiration may bead at the hairline, between the breasts, down the back. Hot flashes can last from one minute to one hour, but most are over in two to three minutes. There may be a chilly sensation for a few moments afterward.

I would like every man and woman to have just one of my hot flashes! First, a sudden, unexplained what's-the-point-of-it-all feeling that lasts only five or ten seconds. I know that within the next thirty seconds I'm going to have a hot flash – waves of heat traveling up my body, perspiration breaking out all over and running down my forehead, a terrible feeling of weakness and exhaustion. I have to sit down or lean against a wall if no seats are available. I'm left with damp clothes (which quickly start to feel cold) and I feel as if I've just finished a hard game of squash – a game I had to give up some years ago. Sometimes I can feel my head pounding during the flash, and sometimes it leaves me with a headache. This can happen from once an hour to four or five times in an hour.

Hot flashes tend to appear during the time that menstrual periods are erratic and to peak during the year of the last menstrual period. They seem to occur most often just before rising and just before bed (6:00 a.m. and 10:00 p.m.), and although many women believe that stress makes the flashes worse, some women find that the frequency and intensity are *not* affected by unusual stress or worry. Such women report equally heavy flashing during times of rest or of relaxation with friends.

The nighttime version of the hot flash is usually more severe. Perspiration may be so profuse that a change of clothing or of bed linen is required. Night sweats that are severe and/or frequent contribute to fatigue and depression. Fortunately, most naturally menopausal women rarely experience flashes this severe.

Dry vagina and urinary distress

With the onset of menopause, there is a tendency for the tissue of the urethra and vagina to thin out and become more fragile. The vagina may also become shorter, and both urethra and vagina become more vulnerable to inflammation and infection. Dry vagina (also known by the medical, but offensive-to-women term, *senile vaginitis*) may mean that a woman's own lubrication is inadequate for pleasurable penile penetration. In extreme cases, the vagina may be so dry that routine movements like walking are uncomfortable. This condition is likely to occur a few years after menopause (usually during the late fifties or early sixties) or as a result of surgical menopause (involving removal of the ovaries).

Recurring cystitis (a burning sensation when urinating) or other urinary problems may occur after hysterectomy as a result of surgery, rather than from natural aging. Damage to the bladder or ureters (tubes running from the kidneys to the bladder) is not uncommon following this operation, particularly if the procedure was done through the vagina – as, for instance, to repair a prolapse.

Even when vaginal or urinary problems are relatively minor, many women complain of frequent urination and a tendency to "leak" when coughing, sneezing, or during orgasm. This is known as *stress incontinence. Urge incontinence* is diagnosed when urine is dribbled on the way to the toilet. Both complaints are common and both are eminently treatable.

Osteoporosis

Osteoporosis means "porous bone" and is a condition that results from excess loss of bone tissue. The onset of osteoporosis is usually painless (which is why it is not listed as a menopausal ailment) and osteoporotic women rarely get warning of its onset, except for periodic backache (often in the lower back) as crush fractures occur. Because the pain eases after a few days and then goes away, few women suspect that a vertebra has collapsed. For most women, the first awareness of osteoporosis follows from a broken bone, often a wrist fracture. This fracture may lead to a series of fractures.

Strictly speaking, osteoporosis is *not* a symptom of menopause, since its onset is based on many factors in addition to menopausal status, most particularly on bone density at about age thirty-five – long before menopause starts. Bone continues to strengthen (that is, become more dense) until the mid-thirties, after which we start to lose bone – at first slowly, then more quickly as we reach the menopause. Five years after the last menstrual period, bone loss slows down again.

It is suspected that osteoporosis comprises a number of different conditions, and there is still a great deal to be known about it. We *do* know, however, that there are at least two types of bone involved: cortical (the hard, shiny outer layer) and trabecular (the honeycomb structure of inner bone or vertebrae). Each type of bone may be affected by a number of factors, and unless you have worked hard to build strong bones during your young adulthood (that is, consumed a lot of calcium and had regular, vigorous exercise), you may have grounds for concern. If you are slight and fair skinned, if you smoke, do not exercise regularly, have never borne or breast-fed a child, and have a history of broken bones in your family, you should take steps to prevent excess loss of bone.

◆

Aside from menstrual irregularity, hot flashes, and dry vagina, a number of ailments, minor and major, are everyday occurrences for many menopausal women. What such complaints have in common is that they are only rarely blamed on menopause, whether in books or articles or in the opinions of most medical practitioners. Indeed, it is sometimes difficult to know whether they are caused by menopause or by aging – a situation that is likely to persist until more solid research is available.

Additional Complaints

If you mention one of these "additional ailments" to your doctor, you are likely to have it dismissed. It very much depends on the person you consult. A knowledgeable physician may take some of these ailments seriously, but it is hard to know which complaint will be attended to and which will be trivialized.

Joint pains

This common ailment often appears before either menstrual irregularity or the first hot flash. When bursitis of the shoulder, tennis elbow, trick knees, aching wrists, sore heels or thumbs, or "funny" ankles trouble a woman, menopause is rarely suspected, but joint aches appear to be linked to the adrenal glands, where cortisone (the substance that keeps joints moving freely) is manufactured. Studies have shown that from one-fifth to one-half of menopausal women experience joint pain at one time or another. It appears to afflict women of all sizes and shapes, whether they engage in regular, vigorous exercise or are somewhat sedentary.

Joint pain is usually restricted to one or two joints and should not be considered in the same class as chronic aches and pains, which may recur for years. Chronic and severe aches and pains may be due to fibromyalgia (explained in detail in Vol. VII, No. 9, of *A Friend Indeed*). Women with fibromyalgia are often mistakenly diagnosed as either arthritic or osteoporotic, although there is no muscle inflammation, damaged tissue, swollen joints, or broken bones. One survey of 100 women with fibromyalgia found that 78 of them had had some kind of surgery to their reproductive organs, suggesting that women who have had a hysterectomy may be more susceptible. It is not likely to happen to you, but those women who have exhausted every other possibility in the search for an explanation for massive aches and pains should know about fibromyalgia.

Migraine

Migraine headaches begin with a spasm in an artery close to the surface of the scalp, on either the left or the right side of the head. Because the headache is confined to one side of the head, a migraine is quite different from a stress headache (which usually comes on slowly) or the "hatband" sensation of a tension headache. Some women will experience bouts of dizziness, strange tingling sensations, or episodes of rapid heartbeat (palpitations); these may be forms of migraine activity *without* the headache. Some women will notice strange "pings" in the back of the head, or what feel like strange surges of blood. It is wise to check out any such symptoms with a doctor, even though these experiences are fairly common.

The relationship between migraines and hormones has been inferred from the onset of common migraine at puberty, the cyclical nature of the symptoms, and the tendency for migraines to disappear (in about 80 percent of cases) during pregnancy and to return again until postmenopause, when, in the majority of cases, they disappear for good.

Some women, however, develop migraines for the first time just prior to menopause. The migraines, whether in the form of headaches or not, occur most commonly during the menstrual period or in the few days following the period. The timing is assumed to be related to low levels of progesterone, but other patterns –

headache at ovulation or just prior to menstruation – may be related to estrogen levels. Or it may be the ratio of estrogen to progesterone that triggers the migraine.

Some women will experience the typical aura (or prodrome) that precedes a migraine, without ever having the headache. The aura is a subjective sensation warning that a migraine is about to start. The aura may take many forms – dizziness, numbness, tingling of the extremities, heightened sensitivity to smells or noise or taste, restlessness, yawning, etc. – but the more common aura is a visual disturbance marked by spots floating before the eyes, then a shimmering outline that gradually obliterates most of the visual field.

Other migraine equivalents are abdominal pain with nausea, vomiting, or diarrhea; acute pain in the chest, pelvis, or extremities; attacks of rapid heartbeat (tachycardia); sudden attacks of dizziness for no apparent reason (benign paroxysmal vertigo); or bloat occurring on a cyclical basis – repeated after a predictable number of days. Each of these symptoms may or may not be accompanied by a headache.

> I experienced severe attacks of vertigo intermittently over a one-year period and they only stopped after a self-imposed regimen of vitamin supplements – Vitamin B_{12}, Vitamin C, and a multiple-vitamin tablet.
>
> The attacks usually came on when I got out of my car in the company parking lot to walk the 150 feet to the entrance. During an attack, if I got up from my chair too quickly, I felt as if I would fall over, and while walking the hallways, I would literally bump into the walls. Now that it is over, I can only attribute the spells of vertigo to stressful situations.

There is no one simple test to establish the presence of a migraine and, even less so, of a migraine equivalent. If you suspect that you are experiencing a migraine equivalent, you might ask your doctor to arrange for medical tests to rule out other possibilities (inner-ear infections, for example, could be responsible for the dizziness). Or you may wish to see a neurologist who specializes in migraine.

Burning-mouth syndrome

Some women experience dry mouth during menopause, a condition that is often aggravated by caffeine and antihistamines, as well as some prescription drugs (e.g., clonidine and some kinds of antidepressants). Because oral tissue is structurally similar to vaginal tissue, dry mouth is thought to be related to the more widely recognized problem of dry vagina. (If dry mouth is accompanied by dry eyes, you should look into the possibility of Sjogren's syndrome.) Others suffer from an extreme case of dry mouth, called burning mouth syndrome (BMS), estimated to affect only 2 percent of the general population, of whom as many as one-fifth may be postmenopausal women. Burning-mouth syndrome often prompts a visit to the dentist with complaints about a chronically burning sensation in the mouth and gums. The cause is not yet understood.

Indigestion, flatulence, bloat

Many women complain about indigestion or flatulence. Some also occasionally experience bloat – the lower torso (waist and belly) swells and remains swollen for two or three hours. This is a very uncomfortable feeling – one that many women remember from pregnancy!

Sleep problems

Changes in sleep habits are very common. Many women find it hard to get to sleep, to stay asleep, or to sleep past the light of early dawn. The average number of hours spent sleeping diminishes from about eight hours at age twenty to about six hours at age fifty and there is a concurrent increase in awakenings. Some of this sleeplessness may be due to hot flashes, which although not severe enough to warrant the term *night sweat* are enough to waken one. Once awakened, many of us head for the toilet. It's hard to know what provokes the wakening – the sensation of warmth or a full bladder.

Most physicians assume that hot flashes cause sleep disruption and that the alleviation of the flashes (using estrogen) will result in restful sleep. Sometimes this is true, but some women experience severe sleep problems that cannot be remedied with estrogen therapy (ET).

Menopause may also be marked by episodes of "air hunger," a sudden and unpleasant sensation of suffocation – gasping for air for a few minutes until it passes. A variation is *sleep apnea*, where breathing stops for a few interminable seconds. Although both sensations last for only a short time, they can be very frightening.

> I have had several unpleasant episodes of sleep apnea over the last two years, two of them severe enough to warrant hospitalization. I really felt quite crazy when I was explaining that I had stopped breathing for a few seconds, but a friend who accompanied the recent Everest expedition had similar symptoms due to the altitude. Unfortunately, my doctor can't offer any help or explanation for this distressing complaint. Neurological tests show nothing wrong.

Weight gain

This is not, strictly speaking, an ailment, since it is so widespread. However, many of us find ourselves being chided by our doctors, and this, together with our own futile efforts to slim, makes it *feel* like a medical problem. Most of us do not eat more than usual. The weight gain is a feature of aging. However, it is hastened by menopause, when the metabolism slows down. Not only are the extra pounds both unexpected and unwelcome, they often accumulate in strange places – on the back, bust, and abdomen – rather than on the hips and thighs.

Skin and hair

Some women complain of a crawling sensation on the skin. The proper medical term for this is *formication*, which is related to the word for ants. It feels as if small ants are crawling on the skin. Patterns of hair growth may change, with underarm hair, pubic hair, and scalp hair thinning out and changing texture, while unwanted facial hair makes an appearance. If scalp hair is thinning (frontal hair loss), a dermatologist or endocrinologist may be needed. The cause is usually assumed to be hereditary male-pattern baldness, which emerges as the male hormones (androgens) assume more importance in our bodies. Other causes of thinning hair may be hypothyroidism, an iron deficiency, or, strangely enough, inadequate stomach acid.

> I am taking estrogen and, so far, have had no problems with it. However, my unhappiness now is that my hair, once curly and pretty, is thinning drastically. Of course, I have changed my hairstyle and tried various "cosmetics." I try to ignore the situation, but am privately terrified. I'm fifty-four years old and want to continue my busy, productive life without the threat of a wig!

Frontal hair loss may also result, paradoxically, from an excess of estrogen – either manufactured in the body (most often by obese women) or taken as estrogen supplements. If scalp hair is thinning too rapidly and in patches, the condition may be *alopecia areata*, which is not related to menopause.

Sensory disturbances

Many women experience what are known as sensory disturbances during menopause, either briefly or for a more extended period of time. They may feel their vision worsening and need a new eyeglass prescription, or they may merely see spots in front of their eyes now and then. Some women report that they hear bursts of sounds more loudly than usual. Some women smell phantom aromas for weeks or months at a time – wood smoke, wet grass, or a dimly remembered scent impossible to identify. Some develop a sensitivity to certain tastes or lose the sense of taste almost entirely. (This latter condition may also be due to use of corticosteroids.) Some women experience *touch impairment*, a sensitivity to being touched, which makes them jumpy, touchy, unable to respond to previously welcome touching by others. These conditions usually are temporary.

Other

In addition, there is a potpourri of annoying physical changes, some of which may be linked to menopause (such as swollen, tender breasts) but most of which may be due to aging. Many women feel overwhelming fatigue. This is probably due to the sheer stress of all the internal bodily changes that are occurring. It is sometimes worsened by interrupted sleep (although one is not necessarily conscious of the interruptions) or thyroid underactivity (hypothyroidism). Some women get "rubber legs," the temporary but frightening sensation that their legs are going to give way underneath them. Some notice weird bruises. It has even been reported that because of hormonal changes menopausal women are more likely to suffer from bad breath!

✦

There is no way of predicting who will experience what ailments, who will have a tough time, and who will have an easy time. Nor is there any magic formula to determine who can and cannot cope. The experience of menopause is as individual as the experiences of pregnancy or childbirth.

If your ailments are more of a nuisance than anything else, you can probably deal with them on your own. Many of the physical ailments of menopause can be managed by alterations in daily routines to eliminate bad habits (smoking and caffeine), to include regular exercise, to add key nutrients to the diet, or to cut back on commitments in order to relieve the stress on your system. Because your immediate interest is in resuming a regular routine, the knowledge that these ailments are likely to be temporary and that they are experienced by many menopausal women will help to restore a sense of control. From this control comes the confidence necessary to deal with the temporary inconveniences of the menopausal years.

If you are feeling ill and unable to deal with day-to-day responsibilities, you should seek professional help. Unfortunately, many doctors do not relate menopause to many of these ailments or, if they do, often do not share this information with their patients. The attitude seems to be that menopausal women are eager to complain and ready to "adopt an ailment" and call it their own. If your ailments are medical, you will need a good physician. More and more doctors are learning to be sympathetic and helpful to their menopausal patients. Shop around for such a doctor. If your menopausal ailments derive from poor nutrition or poor general health, or if they affect your relationships, you may want to consult a holistic health practitioner, a naturopath, a counselor, or a psychotherapist. If you are fortunate, you will find a professional who will work *with* you to find answers to your questions and relief from the most worrisome complaints.

CHAPTER 3

STRATEGIES AND REMEDIES: MEDICAL AND NON-MEDICAL

The decision to seek medical help is often a difficult one. Because menopause has never been a major part of medical studies, many physicians don't know much about it and don't take it seriously. Rather than listening to their patients, they simply tell them to keep busy or to stop thinking about themselves. At the other extreme, gynecologists – the specialists who are *expected* to know about menopause – are often so occupied with women who are truly ill (primarily those who have been hysterectomized) that they view menopause as worse than it really is. Only a few naturally menopausal women have a dreadful time, but because the medical view of menopause defines it as a disease rather than as a normal transition, a specialist may be *too* willing to prescribe powerful drugs.

According to many textbooks on menopause, there are three "symptoms" of menopausal onset: menstrual irregularity, hot flashes, and dry vagina. This is what most doctors look for when you mention menopause. They may also discuss osteoporosis, although osteoporosis is *not* a menopausal complaint, because it is waiting in the wings long before menopause arrives (see chapter 6). However, most doctors won't discuss the menopausal ailments that women complain about to each other. In fact, these ailments are rarely examined in the medical literature. They are covered in the second part of this chapter.

If you view menopause as a natural transition (as I do), you may be interested in ways to make menopause as manageable as possible, including preventive steps and nonmedical ("alternative") remedies. Many women never think of going to a naturopath, nutritionist, chiropractor, or acupuncturist – despite the fact that they have helped many menopausal women. If you are willing to try readily available remedies, you may be able to manage your own menopause without resorting to prescribed medication. Be aware, however, that nonmedical remedies often do not provide immediate relief. The benefits of regular exercise, vitamin or diet supplements, not smoking, etc., take time to be felt. If you decide to experiment with an alternative remedy, be patient. Give each product a fair trial – at least a month or two – before abandoning it. Because more is not necessarily better, it is dangerous to exceed the recommended amounts. If you do your shopping in health food stores, you may find leaflets and publications that often make extravagant claims for various products. Be wary of farfetched claims made by some manufacturers or packagers. Alternative or over-the-counter remedies are not regulated as strictly as prescription drugs.

Menstrual Irregularity

Before you make an appointment with your doctor, it is wise to jot down exactly what is bothering you. If it is menstrual irregularity, keep track of your periods for a few months. Write down the frequency and duration of each period, as well as lightness/heaviness and color of the flow. Because ovulation takes place less and less frequently as we approach menopause, progesterone is sometimes not produced. Because progesterone levels induce menstruation, cycles without progesterone are often longer, with heavier and more profuse bleeding. Cycles that produce such erratic, heavy bleeding can be very bothersome, so it is reassuring to know that this is often a temporary situation preceding true menopause.

Nonprescription remedies

Some women have found relief from a heavy flow by taking Vitamin A supplements (10,000 IUs, or international units, twice daily), by taking over-the-counter antihistamines, or by using a painkiller such as ibuprofen. A controlled study in Britain found that acupuncture often relieves heavy bleeding.

Many women have avoided surgery by keeping records. One woman told me that she had not menstruated for three months. She then had a prolonged period (fifteen days of heavy flow), which might have warranted further investigation. However, her notes on the color and consistency of the flow established that it was actually three periods back to back.

Keep track of when and where you experience any unusual symptoms. Did something happen beforehand that might account for it? Have you had similar experiences in the past?

Medical interventions

Bleeding may sometimes be controlled using naproxen, a mild anti-inflammatory often prescribed for menstrual cramps, or a low-dose contraceptive pill. New guidelines for use of low-dose pills suggest they may be safe for *non-smoking* women to age forty-five. This should of course be confirmed by your doctor. An alternative to the pill is progesterone therapy, sometimes called a *medical D&C*. Synthetic progesterone (usually Provera at 10 mg or 5 mg daily) is administered for ten days; a normal bleed follows when the drug is withdrawn. This therapy can be continued for months until the bleed is negligible, at which point it is inferred that very little estrogen is being produced by the ovaries.

If neither the pill nor the progesterone therapy is effective, a D&C (dilatation and curettage) may be recommended. This procedure often corrects heavy bleeding due to polyps or some forms of uterine fibroids. And newer procedures, which employ a hysteroscope (a fiber-optic device enabling the surgeon to see into the uterus), together with a tiny instrument that fits inside the hysteroscope, permit the doctor to scrape or burn away the lining of the uterus (and the small fibroids that it may conceal). This means sacrificing fertility, but the procedure is minor compared with a hysterectomy and it doesn't entail the after effects of major surgery.

Hot Flashes and Night Sweats

If you experience hot flashes, write down the dates, times, and duration of each. If you suspect that certain situations trigger a hot flash, keep track of them. You may find that you can eliminate or manage heavy flashing by giving up caffeine, reducing or eliminating alcohol and/or certain foods or activities, and choosing different activities at times that seem to bring flashes on. Some women find that they can quickly ward off a hot flash by drinking iced water or by splashing the face with cold water. And, of course, you will find it easier to cope if you dress in layers and wear natural fibers that breathe, rather than synthetics.

One of the least known but most effective ways of minimizing hot flashes is to gain weight. The discomforts that accompany menopause are, to a large degree, caused by the erratic and diminishing production of estradiol (a form of estrogen) by the ovaries and the shift to estrone, an alternative and less powerful form of estrogen. It is useful to know that menopause is *not* the end of estrogen production but rather a time when the body "shifts gears" and begins to use estrogen of a different kind at a different level. Some ovaries continue to produce estradiol fitfully, but successfully, for months or even years. At the same time, androstenedione, a substance produced by both the ovaries and the adrenal glands, is converted into estrone (a secondary form of estrogen) in the adipose (or fatty) tissue of the body. This conversion process becomes more efficient and more effective with age and with a healthy ratio of body fat.

To encourage this shift to estrone production, many nutritionists and geriatricians encourage menopausal women to tolerate a gain of 5 to 7 kg (10 to 15 lbs.) over their "ideal weight." The added weight is also helpful in combating osteoporosis. So don't get *too* upset if a few extra pounds manage to slip onto your frame. The slender women you have always envied may be more affected by hot flashes and may also be more prone to broken bones in old age.

Nonprescription remedies

The most popular products to combat hot flashes are vitamins E and C, evening primrose oil (often recommended for premenstrual syndrome), bee pollen, ginseng, dong quai, and black cohosh.

Vitamin E is measured in international units (100, 200, 400, etc.); the bottled capsules are available in drugstores and health-food stores. Vitamin E is reputed to be effective for one-half to two-thirds of women with hot flashes, but it may be two to six weeks before you notice a difference. Women with diabetes, high blood pressure, or a rheumatic heart condition should take only very small quantities, a maximum of 100 international units daily. *Vitamin E should not be taken by someone on digitalis.* Most women will be comfortable with 600 to 800 IUs, preferably taken after a meal containing some fat. Some advocates of Vitamin E recommend that it be taken with Vitamin C.

Also a popular supplement to combat infection and to counteract the effects of environmental pollution, Vitamin C is measured in grams and is usually recommended in doses of no more than one gram (1000 mg) a day; 500 mg may be sufficient. Too much Vitamin C can cause diarrhea or stomach upset. (Chewable Vitamin C is bad for the teeth.) To make both Vitamin E and Vitamin C more accessible to the body, it is recommended that selenium (25 mcg for each 200 IUs of E) and bioflavonoids (100 mg for each 500 mg of C) also be taken.

If you are unsure of the types and amounts of diet supplements that might help your particular situation, you may want to consult a nutritionist, a naturopath, or a doctor specializing in holistic medicine. If you don't know whom to consult, check with your local health food store to see if they can recommend someone. You can also find names and addresses in the Yellow Pages, or in directories in the many "alternative" magazines sold in health-food stores or on newsstands.

Evening primrose oil (EPO) is another popular remedy for hot flashes. EPO contains gamma-linolenic acid, which is related to prostaglandin activity; prostaglandins are fatty acids involved in the contraction of blood vessels. EPO is promoted for the relief of menstrual cramps, swollen and tender breasts, and hot flashes. Be sure that the product you choose contains a significant amount of gamma-linolenic acid – 40 to 50 percent (there are some very poor quality products on the market). Good EPO is expensive, but women who use it regularly (to relieve PMS, hot flashes, or sleep problems) swear by it, although there are as yet no reputable studies establishing its effectiveness. The recommended dose is two to eight capsules daily. Other sources for gamma-linolenic acid are borage oil and spirulina (blue-green algae).

One of the most exciting developments in the self-management of menopause has been the recognition that phytoestrogens (that is, plant-based estrogens), particularly in the form of soy beans (*glycine max*) and its derivatives, can do much to alleviate the worst menopausal complaints. The benefits of these phytoestrogens can be realized by baking with soy flour (mixed half and half with your regular flour), drinking soy milk, increasing your daily intake of tofu, miso, and other soy products, or by ingesting special soy tablets (e.g., Nutrigenistein) available at health food stores and specialized pharmacies. The joy of soy is that, while adding a modicum of estrogen to the system, it appears to block the action of more powerful estrogens, both endogenous (from the body itself) or exogenous (from other sources). This is partly because phytoestrogens are significantly weaker than laboratory-made estrogens and partly because phytoestrogens lock into estrogen receptors and deflect the activity of proprietary compounds.

A non-soy phytoestrogen product is Promensil which is compounded from red clover.

Ginseng and dong quai (or tan kwai – the spelling varies) are herbs originally imported from the Orient, although most ginseng is now grown here. The ginseng root (*panax ginseng* or *panax quinquefolius*) is recommended for both men and women as a way of increasing the metabolic rate and regaining energy. Ginseng is processed as tablets, capsules, liquid, powder, or tea. People with asthma or emphysema are advised to avoid it because of its histamine-liberating action.

Dong quai (*angelica sinensis*) is often sold as "female ginseng" and is said to have hormonelike properties capable of relieving severe hot flashes. I have found it in tablets and powders. (It is interesting to note that, in China, the use of such herbs and preparations is supervised by pharmacists, who spend six years learning their profession. Medical doctors in China go to school for only five years.)

> A few years ago, I first became aware of occasionally feeling
> hot all by myself, no one else seemed to find it too warm.
> I remember a summer holiday, a 300-mile drive, with all the
> car windows open; I was dressed in two layers of batiste cotton
> and my torso was sheeted with pouring sweat. I had neglected
> to renew my supply of ginseng about a week before the trip.
>   My experience was that so long as I kept ginseng and
> Vitamin E as part of my morning regime, I experienced no hot
> flashes or any other discomfort. The whole business was over
> in three years with not a ripple of reminder since.

Ginseng is also considered to have estrogenic properties, which means that moderation should be the rule. Other sources of estrogen-like substances (phytoestrogens) are found in red clover sprouts, linseed, and soy flour. Diets high in any of these foods will produce a measurable biological response – and may also alleviate hot flashes.

Black cohosh is a herbal remedy that has estrogenic properties and has been found to relieve mild to moderate menopausal complaints for many women. Some of you may make black cohosh tea using flowers (*cimicifuga racemosa*) from your garden. Most women may be glad to learn that Remifemin, a herbal remedy based on black cohosh, originating from and extensively tested in Germany, is now available here and for sale in most natural food stores. It is well worth a try.

Prescription remedies

Clonidine is the generic name of a hypertensive drug (commonly prescribed as Catapres or Dixarit) that is sometimes successful in controlling hot flashes. Because clonidine may contribute to depression, avoid it if you have depressive tendencies. It appears to be more effective if started before flashes become really severe. Even so, it works for only 30 to 40 percent of women who try it. Dixarit is usually prescribed in 0.1 mg tablets, taken once a day. You should feel a difference within two to three weeks if it's going to work. Potential side effects are dry mouth, constipation, headaches, and, occasionally, wild dreams. It is recommended that the medication be discontinued – but always very slowly – after three to six months to reevaluate its use.

Bellergal Spacetabs is another drug sometimes prescribed for hot flashes. A third of the women who try this medication suffer an adverse reaction and must discontinue it. Even when it does work, you should know that Bellergal contains belladonna, phenobarbital, and ergotamine tartrate, and is potentially addictive. For this reason, most health activists feel that it is not suitable for the treatment of menopause.

Occasionally prescribed – for women who cannot or will not take estrogen – are propranolol (Inderal and generics), a beta blocker; the antihypertensive methyldopa (Aldomet and generics); and the dopamine agonist bromocriptine (Parlodel); or a progestin (Provera). In Europe, a number of studies have been published concerning veralipride, an antidopaminergic compound that has been 60 to 80 percent successful in reducing hot flashes. Little interest has been shown in this alternative in this country.

There are many estrogen products available. Still dominating the market is Premarin, a tablet or pill taken once daily (see chapter 5) but there are many other kinds of pills, a vaginal ring, a rub-on gel, and a choice of patches which can be applied twice a week to the thigh, buttock, or abdomen. Not to mention products that can be compounded and tailored to your specific needs. Any estrogen product offers speedy relief of debilitating hot flashes. Although it will not eliminate *all* flashes for *all* women, it is the most effective prescription remedy available. Because the decision about whether to seek or to accept estrogen therapy (ET) remains the central issue for many menopausal women, additional information on use of ET and CHT (combined hormone therapy) is outlined in chapter 5.

If you are considering hormone therapy primarily to relieve hot flashes, you may want to know that:

- Hot flashes last longer for women on hormone therapy.
- Although hot flashes may be alleviated while on hormones, there is a strong possibility that the flashes will return with a vengeance as soon as therapy is discontinued. In other words, hormone therapy masks or postpones hot flashes, rather than eliminating them entirely.
- There are specific contraindications to hormone therapy (reasons why some women cannot or should not take hormones). You should be aware of these in case your doctor is not (see chapter 5).
- There are potential side effects to estrogen and progestins, as there are to any drug. You should know what they are so that you can recognize and deal with them in case they arise.
- Many physicians have personal preferences based on limited experience with certain forms, methods of administration, and dosages (i.e., regimens) of hormone therapy. If you are unhappy with your regimen, you have the right to insist on something different until you find what is appropriate for your unique chemistry.

It is hysterectomized and, most of all, oophorectomized women who suffer from the most severe hot flashes. For these women, and for the small minority of naturally menopausal women who find their hot flashes intolerable, estrogen provides the only certain relief. Most naturally menopausal women suffer as much or more from fatigue due to the physiological stress of constantly adjusting to internal temperature changes and to the embarrassment they feel at having a hot flash in public. If the social stigma of this kind of "flashing" were removed and the embarrassment eliminated, we would all feel better. As more and more women experience the novelty of the hot flash, the day may come when menopausal women will feel free to have hot flashes anywhere, without censure, without shame.

Dry Vagina, Cystitis, Vaginitis

Naturally menopausal women may notice changes in the frequency and pattern of urination while still menstruating, and hysterectomized women may experience urinary distress following surgery.

This is often caused by damage to the bladder or ureters, particularly during vaginal hysterectomy.

Dry vagina is more likely to occur months or years into postmenopause (except when it results from oophorectomy, which produces a sudden drop in estrogen levels). Dry vagina may be detected during regular medical examinations when insertion of the fingers or a speculum is found to be painful. More often, however, a woman notices that penetration by a penis is now uncomfortable.

Dyspareunia, or painful intercourse, continues to be viewed as almost solely a problem of postmenopausal women despite the fact that, according to at least one study, more than 30 percent of women in their thirties experience it occasionally or often. Doctors rarely inquire about painful intercourse when dealing with younger women, but it is a standard question put to women past fifty; this may inflate the estimate of the problem during postmenopause.

Healthy tissue in and around the vagina can be maintained by switching to natural fibers, which allow better air circulation. This means wearing cotton panties and panty hose with cotton crotches or with the diamond-shaped gusset snipped out. Some women prefer stockings with garters. Skirts are preferable to slacks, particularly if the slacks are tight fitting. This may not be important when you're younger, because the labia (lips) around the vagina tend to seal it; with age, the labia become less efficient. If you have a tendency to vaginitis, sitting in a hot tub or Jacuzzi, where bacteria proliferate, can create problems.

> My greatest problem is urinary leakage. Intercourse has
> become uncomfortable for me because of this. It is most dis-
> tressing. The doctors and the specialist I have seen say
> there is nothing that can be done.

Many women notice the need to urinate more frequently, even though they are voiding smaller amounts (urge incontinence) or dribbling involuntarily when coughing, sneezing, or during orgasm (stress incontinence). Both conditions result from the thinning and shortening of tissue in the genitourinary tract and relaxation of the pelvic floor due to aging.

One can adapt to frequent urination, but the best way to prevent leakage is to do Kegel exercises regularly. These exercises, developed by Dr. Arnold Kegel, involve isolating the sphincter muscle which controls urination and strengthening it. If you faithfully practice tightening and loosening this muscle – an exercise that can be done anytime and anywhere – you may find that it not only alleviates incontinence problems, but also enhances the ability to respond sexually.

Kegel Exercises

To locate your pubococcygeal (PC) muscle, simply stop your flow while urinating; it's the PC muscle that contracts to do this. Practice a few times to get the feeling of this muscle. Stop and start urinating at will. Try some stronger and weaker contractions until you can contract this muscle when not urinating. This will help you become familiar with this muscle. You can do your PC exercises anytime you wish; while waiting for a bus or walking down the street, or just after waking. Try them in fitness class when you are working on your abdominals – especially during the pelvic tilt. These two exercises go well together.

Three and Three

Contract your PC muscle for 3 full seconds and then release it for 3 seconds. Repeat 6 times, 3 times a day for a few days. Then repeat 12 times a day for a week.

One and One

Contract your PC muscle strongly for one second and release it for one second. Repeat 20 times, 3 times a day. Speed up the contractions so that you get a "fluttering" feeling here.

Ten and Five

Contract the PC muscle for 10 full seconds, working at holding the intensity of the contraction for the full period of time. Relax for 5 seconds. Repeat 5 times, 3 times a day.

Elevator

As you become more aware of your PC muscle, you will notice that you can feel the difference between your anal and vaginal muscle area. When you start to feel this difference, try the "elevator." Start with an anal contraction (bottom floor) and then move it along the PC muscle into the vaginal area and up to the "top floor." Repeat 6 times, 3 times a day.

Once you have improved your PC muscle tone and can do all of these exercises competently, try maintaining the strength and endurance of your PC muscle by doing your exercises once a day instead of three times. As with most exercise routines, it helps to set aside a specific time and place to ensure that you don't forget.

Source: *Fitness Leader*, September 1983

Nonprescription remedies

Vaginal discharges should be monitored very carefully. Cutting down on dairy products, sugar, and artificial sweeteners may help chronic vaginal infections. Although a douche may give temporary relief, it is not a cure. Nonspecific vaginitis often recurs; in a study of women prone to recurring vaginitis, regular consumption of nonpasteurized yogurt containing acidophilus lactobacillus – 226 g (8 oz.) daily – was found to reduce such episodes by half.

Over-the-counter products are available (and heavily promoted) to relieve vaginitis, but if there is constant irritation, a change in color of discharge, or an unpleasant odor, make an appointment with your doctor to have it properly diagnosed and treated.

To prevent dry vagina, practice regular orgasm (which encourages natural lubrication) and Kegel exercises. If you do not have a regular partner, you might consciously decide to masturbate in order to keep your vagina healthy. If you do have a partner but find intercourse occasionally painful, this may be the time to explore other forms of sexual expression, including oral/genital sex and mutual masturbation.

Many women find intercourse more comfortable with the help of saliva, a water-based lubricant (such as K-Y Jelly or Lubafax), or a Vitamin E suppository. These products are available at the drugstore and can be inserted into the vagina or smeared on the penis prior to penetration. Note that despite all jokes to the contrary, petroleum-based lubricants such as Vaseline are not recommended, because they may damage fragile vaginal tissue. Astroglide, Replens, and

Nutriplens (similar to Replens but with added essential fatty acids and vitamin E) are products that many women find helpful. Of these, Astroglide is the one that has received the most glowing endorsement from the women who have written to me. Phyto-Soya vaginal gel is similar to Replens but with isoflavones and comes in a unit dose applicator similar to that of Replens and Nutriplens. Some women feel ashamed about having to use supplementary lubrication during sex, but many young couples depend on water-based lubricants for comfortable intercourse. Buying a tube of lubricant is not necessarily proclaiming middle-aged inadequacy!

Preliminary evaluations of the new "woman's condom," or vaginal sheath, suggest that this may also be useful in protecting the vagina from direct and painful friction during intercourse.

Since dryness of the vagina is partially due to a change in the chemical environment, some women have had success using natural yogurt internally to restore a healthy vaginal climate. Rosetta Reitz, author of *Menopause: A Positive Approach*, recommends equal amounts of yogurt and a polyunsaturated oil, both as a weekly regimen to keep the vaginal walls elastic, and as a way of lubricating oneself prior to intercourse. Yogurt can be inserted into the vagina using the kind of applicator available with douches or foam spermicide, with a plastic tampon inserter, or with a turkey baster! Because of the consistency of this solution, it is better to be horizontal and to remain horizontal for some time after insertion. And you may want to place a towel under you to protect the bedclothes – or a bearskin rug, depending on your mood!

The tissue outside the vagina, sometimes the whole area around the crotch, may become dry and itchy. If you are already wearing cotton next to the skin, itchiness can often be relieved using "hygienic wipes" – small pads of cotton that are impregnated with witch hazel and glycerin. You can find hygienic wipes at the drugstore, often close to products for hemorrhoid relief. Other products that help to soothe prickly itch are pure shortening and cornstarch. If the itchiness is serious and is felt inside the vagina, you may have developed some kind of dermatitis or perhaps contracted an infection, so consult a dermatologist. As the vaginal tissue thins out, many women become more vulnerable to infections that are not necessarily sexually transmitted.

If you find that you are prone to recurrent bouts of cystitis (bladder infections that produce a burning sensation when urinating), make a habit of drinking large quantities of water. Drinking cranberry or blueberry juice on a regular basis also helps to combat the bacteria responsible for such infections. Avoid using a diaphragm, because it is associated with increased risks of cystitis. If possible, avoid synthetic progesterone (either alone or in conjunction with estrogen), because it may aggravate bladder trouble.

Incontinence is no longer regarded as a corollary of growing older or many pregnancies, although it occurs at a 60 percent higher rate among women who have had a hysterectomy. In addition to practicing Kegel exercises, it is possible to retrain the bladder by timing visits to the toilet: going every hour, then every hour and a half, then every two hours, until you can stay comfortable and dry for three-hour stretches. Some urologists also advocate the use of vaginal cones, which are available in graduated sizes and are held inside the vagina for stipulated periods of time in order to strengthen the pelvic muscles. Others recommend collagen injections to strengthen the sphincter muscle and ensure continence. No matter what the problem, a sympathetic urologist should be helpful in finding a solution.

Prescription remedies

Estrogen cream is commonly prescribed for dry vagina. It is recommended that ten days of oral estrogen precede use of the cream, but this guideline is not universally followed. It is not advisable to take two forms of estrogen, so if you are taking tablets, using the patch, or have had an injection, report this to your doctor. Estrogen cream comes with its own applicator, calibrated in grams, for insertion into the vagina. The recommended dosage on the package is two to four grams daily, on a cycle of three weeks on and one week off. This is often more than most women need.

The most popular estrogen cream is Premarin, which contains 0.625 mg of conjugated estrogen *per gram*. Because estrogen cream is absorbed into the system – with effects on the whole body, not just on the problem area – use of two to four grams of cream daily is potentially equivalent to a daily dose, in oral tablets, of from 1.25 to 2.5 mg, or twice to four times the normal amount. (The amount absorbed is partly dependent on the fragility of the tissue.) Most women find that a fraction of this amount will serve to restore the vagina, although it may take three weeks to reverse the situation. Once the vagina is comfortable again, you can experiment with less frequent use – perhaps two weeks on and two weeks off or, after time, one week of regular use of the cream every month.

The applicator supplied tends to deposit the cream deep into the vagina, but it should also be smeared just inside the opening of the vagina; this is the area that is usually most painful. Estrogen cream, unlike water-based lubricants, is a medication and should *not* be used just prior to intercourse, since it will be absorbed by your partner as well. If you have an intact uterus and use estrogen vaginal cream over a period of months, a course of synthetic progesterone may be advisable every three to six months to make sure that excess endometrial cells are sloughed off.

Antibiotics are often prescribed for cystitis and will usually solve the problem. If the problem recurs and antibiotics seem ineffective, you may be dealing with a case of interstitial cystitis, which requires a different approach. Information about this is available from the Interstitial Cystitis Association. Treatment for vaginitis will depend on the diagnosis but will often involve both the woman and her partner.

For chronic vulvar itch (or vestibulitis – inflammation of the outer part of the vagina), a dermatologist may prescribe a cortisone cream. Although this often solves the problem, cortisone cream can occasionally contribute to *added* thinning of the tissue and merely compound the problem. If you do use cortisone cream, use it sparingly and monitor yourself. (Use a hand mirror to examine the color and texture of the vulvar and vaginal tissue.)

✦

Irregular periods, hot flashes, night sweats, and genitourinary distress are legitimate concerns that you may wish to discuss with your doctor. You deserve a sympathetic and supportive hearing, and since these complaints are commonly associated with menopause, you will probably receive some counseling about the advantages and disadvantages of medication.

Other menopausal complaints are not taken quite so seriously, despite the publicity given to menopause. This may be because these ailments are often not relieved by ET or CHT. If it is assumed that menopause ailments are caused by an estrogen deficiency, it is difficult to believe that supplementary estrogen cannot alleviate the full range of complaints. But, whether we like it or not, this is true.

Joint Pain

If you experience joint pain, you should check with a doctor. If tests for arthritis are negative, however, chances are that the pain is associated with menopause and is a temporary nuisance. Many women have found that extra Vitamin B_6 (1.5 to 2.0 mg daily) or combinations of Vitamin C and cod liver oil (Vitamin D) relieve the ache. Your doctor may suggest a cortisone shot (which masks the pain without relieving the cause), or you may consult a physiotherapist about appropriate exercises to ease the stiffness and/or pain. However, for all those women (including myself) who have been diagnosed with frozen shoulder, or tennis elbow, or housemaid's knee, or carpal tunnel syndrome, or heel spurs, or sore thumbs, or any other affliction that is more annoying than incapacitating, you might just want to wait it out. It may just go away.

Migraine

Migraine headaches have been a bane of mine for years, but they have had no regularity. Mine fall into the "common" category. Sometimes I feel they are caused by food allergies, cosmetics, smoke, and stress. I usually wake up in the morning with a migraine, don't have any warning symptoms, and the bad ones last three days, with nausea, vomiting (which usually provides relief), a peculiar metallic taste in my mouth, and a feeling of general malaise.

Countless experiments have been conducted on alleviating migraine with hormonal preparations – estrogens, progesterones, combinations of these and other hormones. But because so many young women suffer their first migraine after starting on "the pill" and because the hormonal status responsible is not yet understood, migraine sufferers are generally discouraged from taking any form of supplementary hormones. Since the blood vessels in the head are dilated during migraine, there is concern that hormone use might promote blood-clot formation; these clots might loosen, be carried into the brain, and cause a stroke.

Migraines can be triggered by such things as loss of sleep, over-sleeping, fasting (low blood sugar), falling barometric pressure, glaring sunshine, and flickering fluorescent or strobe lights. Many migraine sufferers (the correct term is migraineurs) cannot adequately process foods containing certain types of amines, although the headache may not start for hours after eating the foods responsible. Some of the most common culprits are aged cheese (cheddar), chocolate, vinegar, sour cream, yogurt, yeast products, nuts, onions, citrus fruits, bananas, pork, caffeine-rich beverages, cured cold meats, and alcohol. This reaction to food is not an allergy in the common sense of the term; the amine-containing substance can only rarely be isolated using standard allergy tests.

More mysterious than the migraine headache is the migraine equivalent, a disturbance that appears to be generated in the same way as the headache but without the ache. Migraine equivalents may be merely the aura (prodrome) of the headache – spots in front of the eye, disturbed vision, dizzy spells – or may manifest themselves in effects on one side of the body – a pain down one side, a glowing red ear, a throbbing or dull ache in the abdomen. The variations are many, but these weird experiences seem to become more common as menopause approaches. It may take determination and persistence to find a well-informed neurologist who can offer support and understanding.

Other migraineurs may have yeast infections (systemic candida albicans, an overgrowth of a normal flora found in the body) or temporomandibular joint syndrome (faulty articulation of the hinged joint of the jawbone; a condition that may cause, in addition to headache, dizziness or ringing in the ears). It is suspected that a tendency to migraine may also result from a major trauma in childhood, such as physical or sexual abuse.

As soon as a migraine starts, the most effective therapy is to lie down in a quiet, darkened room. Other preventive measures are splashing the face with cold water or stepping into a steamy, hot shower (to dilate the blood vessels in the head) and then gradually switching to cold water (to contract the blood vessels). Not an inviting prospect!

Many migraineurs have learned to control their headaches with variations of biofeedback, relaxation therapy, and visualization. Biofeedback is usually taught at a headache or pain clinic and frequently includes exercises in progressive relaxation. One form of biofeedback teaches the person to raise the temperature of the hands using visual imagery (that is, imagining one's hands in the sun or dipped in a basin of warm water). As the hands warm up, the headache starts to go away. Another visualization technique is to see the headache contained in a glaring light bulb. Then, by using the full power of imagination, the light bulb is gradually dimmed. All such techniques require supervised practice initially but, once mastered, frequently provide an effective way to control migraine and, at the same time, to break the reliance on drugs.

Today more credence is given to the very real pain experienced by many migraine sufferers. If you have exhausted other possibilities and are unwilling to rely on drugs for relief, it might be worthwhile to inquire about a pain clinic at your nearest large hospital.

Nonprescription remedies
Over-the-counter preparations – acetaminophen (Atasol, Tylenol) or aspirin – may be useful if taken immediately at onset and/or for mild migraines. Preparations containing codeine are not recommended because they are addictive and may cause nausea or vomiting. In Britain, research at the University of Nottingham has demonstrated that the herb feverfew (*tanacetum parthenium*) has the ability to ward off or reduce the severity of a migraine. Because feverfew is not available in standardized doses, use of this herbal remedy requires a bit of experimentation.

Prescription remedies

The standard prescription drug is ibuprofen (Motrin, Amersol, etc.). In about 50 percent of cases, ergotamine tartrate (Ergomar, Gynergen, etc.), taken immediately at onset, wards off or shortens the migraine. Ergotamine is available in tablet form, in an inhaler, as a suppository, or by injection. Variations are ergot-and-caffeine (Cafergot), and belladonna-ergot-and-phenobarbital (Bellergal Spacetabs). Frequent use of any ergot preparation is dangerous. Migraineurs who use ergot must remain under medical supervision to prevent overuse and rebound headaches, which may be even worse than the original migraine.

A prescription drug is succinate of sumitriptan, marketed as Imitrex, and available in pills or injections. Although it is very expensive, one pill or self-administered injection may be enough to halt a migraine in its tracks. There is some concern, however, about adverse effects (chest pains, breathlessness), and these will have to be investigated before Imitrex can be fully accepted.

Migraines that occur more often than two or three times a month can be treated with preventive drugs. Beta blockers are often prescribed, but beware of side effects. Propranolol (Inderal), for instance, often causes restless sleep with frequent awakenings. Calcium blockers, anti-inflammatories, and antidepressants can also be employed in an effort to prevent migraines. In fact, the wide range of drugs used in an attempt to halt migraines is an indication of the enormous puzzle that migraine poses. Any of these medications has potential side effects. None should be taken for more than a few months.

Burning-Mouth Syndrome

Four years ago, in the middle of the afternoon, my mouth caught fire. And it remained that way for three years! For a few hours, I put it down to something I ate. After a few days, I became suspicious that it might be something more serious. After a few weeks, I saw my doctor.

Over the months since, I have seen many doctors – a family physician, dermatologist, allergist and dentist. No one could diagnose the problem. To relieve it, I tried sucking on Popsicles, ice cubes, mints, or chewing gum – anything wet or cold. A year later, I heard on the news that a mysterious disease had doctors baffled. Patients were complaining of a burning mouth and tongue. It was now recognized as a genuine disorder. I felt vindicated! The symptoms persisted for another year. but I took comfort in the fact that I was not alone.

Although we know that dry mouth can result from too much caffeine or too many antihistamines, burning-mouth syndrome is harder to treat. Sucking on ice cubes or peppermint lozenges and drinking cold water are the usual responses to this syndrome, but the only lasting relief has been found to be massaging the gums. Because it is assumed that this condition is related to changes inside the vagina (the tissue involved is similar), studies have been done using Vitamin E oil or estrogen cream as a "massage agent." Both appear to be equally effective; it is the massage that seems to make the difference. The only good news about burning-mouth syndrome is that it has been treated successfully with acupuncture, it appears to spontaneously disappear after a while, and it is now being taken more seriously by researchers in medicine and dentistry.

Indigestion, Flatulence, Bloat

During middle age, many persons (both men and women) develop lactose intolerance and find milk and milk products (with the exception of yogurt) difficult to digest. For some, garlic, or green pepper, or cucumber may suddenly create problems. Foods high in fat often cause heartburn. All of this is very common and un-doubtedly due more to aging – and to changes in the amount and efficacy of gastric acid – than to menopause. However, such prob-lems often show up for the first time during the menopausal years. Perhaps you should keep a log of the foods you eat so that you can do some detective work.

If you notice excess gas after drinking milk or eating cheese, you may want to buy a lactase enzyme. It is sold in drugstores and health-food stores, in liquid or tablet form. When added to milk, which must then sit for a few hours, it predigests the lactose. (Pretreated milk is also available but is more expensive.) You can then have the benefit of the calcium in milk without the problem of indigestion. Yogurt, although technically a milk product, is often easier to digest than milk or cheese and can help the body to digest other foods high in lactose.

In addition, foods high in potassium – bananas, apricots, tomatoes, or orange juice – can relieve excess gas and can also help to reduce the risk of stroke! Papaya tablets or activated charcoal (both available at health-food stores) also prevent that terrible gassy feeling.

> Gas problems have been an embarrassment for several years. Initially I put the blame on irregular hours, eating habits, diet, what have you. I tried eliminating certain foods and adding others. Meat seemed to be hard to digest, so I tried some papaya tablets. When the papaya helped somewhat, I got a stronger version. It solved my problem with flatulence completely.

> Bloat is somewhat of a mystery. It may very well occur as a result of eating some of the foods mentioned, but it also seems to happen for no reason at all. I vividly remember surreptitiously unzipping my jeans at the dinner table one evening and then finding, to my consternation, that I could not zip them up again! My waist size had suddenly increased by two to three inches, although it was back to normal the next morning. Keep track of what you eat, but remember that bloat is fairly common and that these episodes disappear with time.

Sleep Problems

As we age, we tend to need less and less sleep. The need men have for sleep seems to diminish gradually. Many women, however, suddenly find themselves wide-awake in the middle of the night or waking regularly with the first light of dawn. Room-darkening shades or blind-folds are often effective. A glass of warm milk before bed also helps, because warm milk releases tryptophan, an amino acid that is an effective and mild sleep inducer. Antihistamines that relieve motion sickness (dimenhydrinate or Gravol) or cold symptoms (Dristan, Contac-C, Chlor-Tripolon, etc.) may also induce drowsiness.

Regular exercise improves the quality of sleep. Many women find that a walk after dinner will help them to fall asleep more easi-ly. Practitioners of yoga can teach their bodies to relax, since deep breathing invites sleep. Some women find progressive relaxation helpful. Audiotapes that give instructions in this technique are available from sleep clinics and clinical psychologists, or through advertisements in magazines dealing with health and well-being.

Although sleep apnea is more common among men, if you awak-en frequently gasping for breath or if you begin to snore very loudly, you may want to be checked at a sleep lab (or clinic) at your local hospital. Or you may find an experimental psychologist interested in this problem; try calling the psychology department of your local university.

Routine sleeplessness is a temporary aggravation of menopause. It helps to realize just how much can be accomplished on very little sleep. I hear from women who bake, or read, or write letters, or watch old movies for an hour or two in the middle of the night. Yet they put in a full day's work every day! The stamina of the midlife woman is admirable.

Prescription remedies

If sleeplessness due to hot flashes or night sweats leads to intolerable fatigue, a short course of estrogen may help. ET may contribute to more restful sleep by allowing you to fall asleep more quickly (the period of time known as "sleep latency") and adding to the ratio of dream sleep. The amount of dream sleep is one criterion of quality sleep – sleep that leaves you feeling refreshed. In fact, sleepers who are deprived of dream sleep exhibit abnormally high levels of anxiety.

Sleeping pills, on the other hand, reduce the amount of dream sleep. If you cannot or will not take estrogen and depression is not a problem, you may want to ask your doctor to prescribe a mild tranquilizer. Tranquilizers are not as soporific as sleeping pills and are less likely to produce a "drugged" feeling the next morning. But remember, tranquilizers are depressants and can be addictive, so don't use them unless you know that they will be a "sometime" thing – once every ten days or two weeks. If you know that you have addictive tendencies, don't use them. If you find you are using them more often, flush them away.

Weight Gain

Even when one is aware of how extra weight can benefit bones and alleviate hot flashes, it is hard to accept living with a weight gain of 4.5–7 kg (ten to fifteen pounds). If weight soars beyond this extra cushion of fat – to 20 percent more than ideal weight, the threshold of obesity – one is inviting a host of medical problems. The only solution to permanent weight loss is a long period of sensible eating and a loss of no more than two pounds a week. Prolonged diets have the advantage of inducing improved eating habits, including a sharp cutback in alcoholic beverages. Weight gain is discussed more fully in chapter 8.

Other

Skin and hair

Dry skin and dry hair are often improved by regular exercise, which seems to lubricate the system generally. Dry skin benefits from products that use a petrolatum or lanolin base. It is not necessary to buy expensive products. The "crawling skin" sensation can be relieved by ET, but I have heard from a number of women who have successfully used homeopathic remedies for this complaint. Hair may appear to thin out as the hair grays and the texture changes. And hair may also thin either as a result of excess estrogen in the system or as a result of the influence of androgens. Some women find that starting estrogen supplements halts hair loss, whereas others find that stopping estrogen (or losing a substantial amount of weight) achieves the same effect. If you are convinced that you are losing an inordinate amount of hair, you might want to consult a specialist, who may prescribe spironolactone, an antiandrogen that is often used to treat women with excess body hair but that, paradoxically, often helps to restore hair lost at the front of the head. Because spironolactone has powerful, often unpleasant side effects and because long-term effects are unknown, milder remedies – such as a herbal rinse made of stinging nettles – may be a wiser choice. Minoxidil (Rogaine) is being strongly promoted to relieve hair loss, but it's expensive, takes about eight months of daily application to determine its effectiveness, works for only 30 to 40 percent of those who try it, and must be used for life. Side effects include itching and prickling, headaches, dizzy spells or light-headedness, and irregular heartbeat. It is also too early to know about possible long-term effects.

Allergies and sensitivities

Despite the fact that any other period of hormonal fluctuation – puberty, pregnancy, and childbirth – is acknowledged to be a time when allergies and sensitivities arise or sometimes go into remission, there is no documented evidence that this is also true for menopause. However, the anecdotal evidence – hundreds of letters – that I have received convinces me that this is a fairly common occurrence.

Be alert to newly developed sensitivities. I have found that my eyes run when the wind is cold – a form of rhinitis (inflammation of the nose) that may have something to do with urban pollution but that certainly started during menopause. Other women report that they now have a bad reaction to cigarette smoke. Some women have found that certain foods – wheat, for instance – add to a sense of fatigue.

◆

My problem is one I've never heard anyone else mention – bruises. They are large or small and resemble the type of surface bruise incurred when you bump yourself. However, I'm sure I haven't bumped myself and they seem to get worse when my flashes are more frequent.

If you experience one of the more unusual ailments – tachycardia (rapid heartbeat), mysterious bruises, attacks of dizziness, "rubber legs" – keep track of when and where it occurs. Tachycardia can be due to mitral valve prolapse (and should be checked out with a cardiologist), but if no cause can be found for it, relief may sometimes be found by adding magnesium to the diet. Dizziness can be a migraine equivalent. In all cases of suspected menopausal ailments, try to figure out if something happened in the past that might account for it. Have you had any similar experiences before? What have you done to try to make yourself feel better? Your complaint may or may not be taken seriously, but a conscientious doctor will order tests to rule out conditions that might cause the same or similar complaints. You may have to do without firm professional assurance that the ailment is related to menopause, but you may be relieved to find that you are generally healthy.

One of the most common remedies offered to menopausal women is the tranquilizer, a drug that is both addictive and a depressant. With the sole exception of sleeplessness, which can be relieved by the infrequent use of a mild tranquilizer, none of the physical ailments discussed in this chapter calls for a prescription for alprazolam (Xanax), lorazepam (Ativan), or diazepam (Valium). Doctors may offer a prescription not because they know it will alleviate a particular complaint, but because they know that patients expect to leave with a prescription. It is the concluding ritual of the appointment and a way of validating the patient's complaint. If your doctor can only suggest tranquilizers, you may want to find another physician or consult with another kind of health practitioner.

CHAPTER 4

PSYCHOLOGICAL
AND SEXUAL
EFFECTS

This chapter deals with psychological and sexual effects of menopause separately from other ailments not because they are any less important than physical ailments, but because they require a different approach. Many women who freely admit to hot flashes turn suddenly shy when talking about panic attacks or loss of sexual desire. The causes of each of these may be similar – a temporary biochemical disturbance – but less is known about the psychology and sexuality of menopause. Because the precise hormonal interactions are so poorly understood, no standard diagnosis or treatment has been formulated.

Physicians are thus often ill-equipped to conduct discussions of mood swings, anxiety, panic attacks, and depression. When they refer their patients to a psychologist or psychiatrist, the patient feels that her problem is being redefined as emotional or mental, when *she* believes that it is due to stress on the *body*.

In the same way, sexual problems involve not only the physical responses of the woman, but also the whole complex of attitudes and feelings of the woman and her partner. If physicians are ill-equipped to handle psychological complaints, they are even more uncomfortable with sexual questions. It helps to know that although some psychological and sexual effects require medical expertise, others can be solved through increased self-knowledge or better communication, and that both of these can often be facilitated by a qualified therapist.

Psychological Problems

Memory lapses

Menopausal forgetfulness is not something that most doctors care to discuss, nor do most women wish to bring it up. Many of us joke, somewhat uneasily, about the onset of Alzheimer's disease, although most Alzheimer victims apparently are not aware of their failing memories. However, *we* feel the lack, and for many women, part of the frustration is having this faltering memory brought to their attention. Women have traditionally remembered the birthdays, the items needed at the store, the names of casual acquaintances. Now we feel we are letting others down. Again, there is a sense of loss. Of all the psychological effects of menopause, forgetfulness is probably the most common. We are told that this is due to age, that we have too much on our minds, that it is due to stress, and that men have it too. We are also directed to articles that teach us how to remember – mnemonic exercises to help us remember names or items on a list.

> Last year I could go to the supermarket and remember ten items without a list. This year I walk upstairs to get *one* thing and forget why I went upstairs. Last year I knew the first names of all the wives of my husband's club members, whom I see once every six months; this year, I remembered the names of two. Yesterday I put the bread in the freezer and the ice cubes in the bread box. Today I'm buying another notebook to keep yet more lists.

Some nutritionists believe that memory lapses are partly due to a deficiency of a particular kind of lecithin (a phospholipid found in eggs and seeds); other experts say that the body manufactures all the lecithin we need. Preliminary studies tell us that removal of the ovaries can result in perceptible differences in the ability to concentrate and to retain information. Such differences are not so noticeable among naturally menopausal women. And the deficits that *do* exist are not significant. Even at its worst, menopausal forgetfulness is no worse and no different from what would be considered within the range of normal in any other context or with any other group.

(By the way, despite news items to the contrary, estrogen therapy [ET] has *not* been found to improve memory in healthy menopausal women, although it has some small effect on women who suffer from memory loss after surgery involving removal of the ovaries. Nor has it been proven effective in significantly delaying, preventing, or alleviating Alzheimer's disease.) Menopause may be a time for women to abandon their self-imposed role of "memory bank" for the boss, husband, and children. Despite rumors to the contrary, there is no demonstrated relationship between menopausal forgetfulness and the onset of Alzheimer's disease. The ability to concentrate, together with attention span and memory, appears to improve after the worst of menopause.

Anxiety

Many women find that the onset of menopause makes them more anxious. Chores that were once routine become fraught with worry. A teacher is suddenly self-conscious in front of her class; an executive is filled with self-doubt prior to a routine presentation to a client; a hostess worries herself sick about a run-of-the-mill dinner party. Such women are victims of free-floating anxiety, which afflicts many women as they enter menopause. The anxiety does not seem linked to any particular event; it is simply there. What was once considered new and fun becomes worrisome, even frightening. Many women force themselves to take on new challenges, and at the same time feel great empathy for women who find that routine chores are almost more than they can handle. Like many other facets of menopause, these flurries of anxiety – particularly when a woman is faced with the new and untried – are likely to be temporary. It may be some comfort to think about the countless menopausal women lying in bed at night, self-consciously reviewing their stupidities of that day – an activity they had intended to give up at age fifteen!

One problem with anxiety is that it is so relative. Some women are anxious all the time and, although probably thought of as high-strung, appear to function adequately, if not serenely. What distin-- guishes true neuroticism from normal neuroticism (and we're all neurotic about something) is its degree and duration. Anxiety becomes debilitating when it seriously hampers one's regular activi- ties over a long period of time. Persons who make radical changes to established routine in order to avoid stressful situations and who maintain this avoidance behavior for months are exceeding ordinary anxiety. If the disorder persists, it may become phobic, and profes- sional help should be sought. This occurs only rarely.

For most of us, it is comforting to know that the sense of anxiety is shared, that many other women are feeling the same way, and that, like many of our physical woes, it will go away in time. Meanwhile, perhaps we should order our nearest and dearest to refrain from expressions such as, "Don't worry," "Just relax," or (the one I hate) "Lighten up, will you?" We will stop worrying and start relaxing when we are no longer feeling so anxious. And we will let the Pollyannas around us know when this happens!

Irritability

Irritability is even more visible than anxiety. We get angry about things that never bothered us before. We shake with rage over a tri- fling matter. The puzzlement we feel about our behavior is often rein- forced by puzzled looks on the faces of close friends, coworkers, or family members. It is worth considering whether irritability is more of a problem for you (the woman) or for those close to you. Many women are more concerned about the effect they have on others than they are about themselves. This leads to a situation where a woman seeks help or accepts medication for the benefit of those who tell her that she is not "herself." Unwilling to ask others to adjust to this newly willful person, the woman may accept some sort of chemical help (usually a tranquilizer) to restore her amiability.

While it is true that menopausal women can be unusually "bitchy," they can also be unusually assertive, creative, and self-pro- tective. It is *not* that a particular incident now irritates when it never irritated before. It's just that they are not willing to put up with that particular irritant one more time. It may be that they're not feeling well (and therefore it irritates more); it may be something that has always been vexing and it is now time to speak out about it. Because menopause makes us sharply conscious of aging, we are more aware of the life we have left to live, and often superconscious of the annoying traits and behaviors of those around us. We may never have mentioned it before, but the prospect of living with it (whatever "it" is) any longer may be intolerable.

Looked at in another way, many women come into their own at menopause. They have put the needs of others first for many years. Menopause may be the trigger that makes women demand their fair share for the first time. Sometimes this newfound assertiveness is channeled into a new enterprise, whether hobby or work. The sense of impatience, of too much to do and not enough time to do it, persuades women to return to school, to take up new challenges, to give up chores and responsibilities that have chafed or bored. There are many positive aspects to this "irritability."

> In order to survive, I needed blocks of unfractured time
> and private space. Our children usually have rooms of their
> own; our parents have living space of their own. We mothers
> and wives may lay partial claim to a "master bedroom"
> (and hear what I am saying because we use words without
> thinking). A woman I spoke to not long ago said that what
> she wants is to find a dark closet somewhere and get some
> peace. I suggested a more daring approach – her own room
> in the house! And not a sewing room or a corner of the
> living room either!
>   When I found myself sighing and sometimes crying in
> the bathroom (often after having waited to get in), I knew
> I was in deep trouble.

The standard "remedy" for anxiety and irritability is a tranquilizer. If you accept a prescription, be sure that you do so for your *own* benefit, not merely to pacify those around you. Be aware also that it is potentially addictive and a depressant. If you are already feeling depressed, as well as anxious and irritable (a common situation), the tranquilizer will make you feel *more* depressed.

Panic attacks

After turning fifty, I suddenly found myself drenched in perspiration while out shopping, experiencing some very nasty
dizzy spells and feelings of unreality, and I began to dread the
daily trips to the supermarket. After a while, I began drop-
ping my purchases and making a beeline for the nearest
exit and home. The *worst* thing I could have done, of course,
as counseling has since taught me! But try telling that to
a person having a bad panic attack. They wouldn't stay
around long enough to listen to you, let alone heed your
good advice!

Frankly, I am convinced that the chemical and hormonal imbalance that menopause brings about *does* play a
very large part in upsetting our equilibrium. Some of us
manage to muddle through somehow without falling apart
at the seams. Others become so afraid that they become
housebound.

Panic attacks, a more focused form of anxiety – and, fortunately,
relatively rare – involve the body as well as the mind. During a panic
attack, adrenaline rushes into the bloodstream, the heart pounds,
the palms of the hands sweat, and breathing becomes quick and shallow. Although the attack is undoubtedly caused by some sudden
change in brain chemistry, the mind seems to seize on some*one* or
some*thing* as a cause. Suddenly, out of nowhere, we imagine a terrible accident about to happen to a loved one, or something unspeak-
ably embarrassing that we are about to do, such as faint or fall over.
It is only after the panic abates that we realize that the pounding
heart and quick breathing came *first*, that the situation itself did not
cause the panic attack.

Many menopausal women deal with panic attacks by breathing
slowly and deeply and by counting, singing, whistling, or reciting
nursery rhymes (anything that drives away negative thoughts). Some
women carry a small brown paper bag to breathe into, which often
wards off hyperventilation – abnormally quick, shallow breathing. If
the panic attacks are very severe or the recurrence restricts activity

in any way, it is time to get help. A good psychotherapist can provide the tools to enable you to get past this kind of block.

It would be helpful to have an explanation for these bizarre menopausal episodes, but so far, no one has been able to trace the effects of brain chemistry on specific behaviors such as these. Menopause, by itself, may be a source of stress for the body, and this stress often adds to existing stress – stress imposed by the burden of commitments in the roles of wife, daughter, mother, housekeeper, worker, friend. In other words, it is probably not menopause *itself* that induces anxiety (or irritability or panic attacks) but rather the extra, added stress of menopause that is unbearable.

I have come to the conclusion that the mind tries to give a name or substance to its fears when attempting to deal with free-floating anxiety, and that just about anything will do. I am now fifty-six and panic far more easily than I ever did before middle age and the onset of "the change." To be honest, in the past few years, I find myself panicking over so many stupid little things that in earlier years I would have never given a second thought to.

I also experience spells of great sadness at times and weep for no good reason. Sometimes there just seems to be an awful feeling of doom, as if something dreadful were about to happen. Just as quickly as these feelings come, they disappear.

Depression

Of all the psychological effects of menopause, the most dreaded is undoubtedly depression. Despite the fact that menopausal women are *less* likely to suffer from clinically diagnosed depression than are much younger women (particularly mothers of young children), depression continues to be a bugaboo. Not only are women frightened about being depressed, they're ashamed to admit that they *are* depressed. Somehow this condition doesn't seem fitting for a "mature" woman in her forties or fifties. There is also the stigma of depression: depressed women have traditionally been treated as if they were personally responsible. They "didn't have enough to do" or "thought about themselves too much." Although these destructive attitudes linger (it's called "blaming the victim") more and more we see that *some* women, for no known reason, *do* get depressed at menopause. This is much more likely to happen if menopause is surgically induced, or if the woman has experienced a depression at some other stage in her life, but it also happens to women who believe they have absolutely no reason to feel depressed. Menopause affects brain chemistry, depression results from a temporary imbalance in brain chemistry, and depression is self-limiting. In other words, a depression will go away whether you seek help or not. For most of us, the biggest struggle is to acknowledge depression – either in oneself or in a friend.

Menopausal depressions almost never involve manic or bipolar depression – a depression followed by a period of manic activity and energy and widely recognized as a genuine mental illness. It is rather a depression characterized by fatigue and an absence of a sense of purpose or of worth. According to the *Diagnostic and Statistical Manual of Mental Disorders*, 4th edition:

> The essential feature of a Major Depressive Episode is a period of at least two weeks during which there is either depressed mood or the loss of interest or pleasure in nearly all activities. ... The individual must also experience at least four additional symptoms drawn from a list that includes changes in appetite or weight, sleep, and psycho-motor activity; decreased energy; feelings of worthlessness or guilt; difficulty thinking, concentrating, or making decisions; or recurrent thoughts of death or suicidal ideation, plans or attempts.

Menopausal depression has been found to be abnormally high among women who have had hysterectomies and oophorectomies (occurring in from 55 to 75 percent of cases and peaking two years after the operation). However, depressed women are also more likely to *report* severe menopausal symptoms (to a clinic or to their doctors), which may be why depression is so often linked with menopause. It is often hard to know which came first, the depression or the menopause.

> I am forty-seven and was not going through menopause
> until hysterectomy completely devastated me a year ago.
> I knew nothing of menopause – had had no hot flashes or
> depression. Now I can really relate to other women who are
> suffering these symptoms. I have had a terrible year. I find
> the depression worse than anything else. I wake up each
> morning with a silent prayer, "Please, God, let me have one
> good day so I can bear the rest." The odd good day keeps me
> going. I have wonderful friends and a husband who is loving
> and caring. If it were not for his tender understanding,
> I would never get through.

There is no real agreement about the cause of depression, but there are two main theories. The first is that depression results from a reaction to the biological or social facts of being a woman. Women suffer from depression in numbers estimated to be from two to six times greater than the rate for men. Depression may be "rage turned inward": women may experience depression because they do not act out their anger in the same way that men do. Instead of venting resentment or hostility in verbal or physical ways, women transform it into guilt, anxiety, or depression. An archaic term for menopausal depression, *involutional melancholia*, means an inward-turning sadness.

The depressed menopausal woman may be mourning – mourning the loss of reproductive ability, mourning the babies she never had, mourning the opportunities missed, mourning her loss of attractiveness. Or she may feel depressed because she has lost the socially valued role of mother (which often coincides with menopause) and must now confront the prospect of old age. There is a mourning, but this is not so much a mourning of reproductive ability as a mourning for the social role that had defined that woman's place in her world. In her book *Women and Madness*, Phyllis Chesler says, "Women are in a continual state of mourning – for what they never had – or had too briefly, and for what they can't have."

These explanations for midlife depression are all rooted in circumstances particular to the female. When we look at woman's role in this society, at the shockingly high rates of sexual and spousal abuse directed at females, we can understand how valid are women's deep-seated resentments, which may show themselves as depression.

There is also a biochemical basis for some kinds of depression. Postpartum depression (the kind of depression that follows childbirth, whether a temporary "blues" or a more long-standing condition) is assumed to be caused by an imbalance in hormones affecting brain chemistry (or brain chemistry that affects hormones). A woman who has just given birth moves into a high-risk category for depression, as does the woman who has had a hysterectomy, whether or not the ovaries are left. No equivalent surgery (appendectomy, gallbladder surgery, etc.) produces the risk of depression that follows from trauma (natural or induced) to the female reproductive organs. Logically, then, menopause *may* (not *will*) induce depression in a minority of women as a result of some kind of biochemical effect. In real life, of course, it is often difficult to distinguish between a depression that is biochemically caused and one that is triggered by social experience, present or past.

Some women fight off depression with a combination of supplementary Vitamin B_6 and a lot of exercise. Physical exertion has been found to change brain chemistry and to promote a more optimistic attitude.

The herbal remedy St. John's Wort (*hypericum perforatum*) has been extensively tested and found effective in cases of mild to moderate depression (*not* severe or clinical depression). It is available in capsules in drugstores and health food stores; allow six weeks for it to take effect.

If this is not enough, you need someone to talk to. You should consult a clinical psychologist, a psychotherapist, or a psychiatrist. Psychiatrists are medical doctors who can prescribe drugs, whereas psychologists and psychotherapists may not have this right. To see a psychiatrist in private practice, you will need a referral from your regular health professional. The alternative is to use the outpatient psychiatric services at your local hospital or to speak to your nearest mental health association. Psychologists and many psychotherapists advertise; if you cannot or do not wish to get suggestions or referrals from friends or other health professionals, check with trained counselors at a nearby school or university. Counselors know the best therapists in the community.

Whether you are dealing with a psychiatrist, psychologist, or psychotherapist, you should have some positive feelings about his or her competence and personality during the first visit. If not, try someone else.

You may also be offered medication – either by your regular doctor, by a psychologist (working with a medical doctor), or by a psychiatrist. The first choice may be estrogen, although the *Physician's Desk Reference* (46th ed.) tells us that "there is no adequate evidence that estrogens are effective for nervous symptoms or depression which might occur during menopause and they should not be used to treat these conditions."

It has been effectively demonstrated that menopause does not *cause* depression. What menopause may do is cause an intolerable amount of internal, physiological, and uncontrollable stress that, when added to the other stresses of the midlife woman, makes it impossible to cope. The work of John and Sonja McKinlay, and of Susan Ballinger, clearly shows that it is the *other* stresses that cause the problem. Estrogen therapy may be useful in a small minority of cases, perhaps because it relieves night sweats, allows a woman to sleep better, and thus enables her to cope with the other stresses. But in the vast majority of cases, estrogen becomes a way to avoid dealing with problems aside from menopause.

The other "solution" available by prescription is tranquilizers, which will just make a woman more depressed. For authentic depression, antidepressants are preferable. They may stimulate the brain to produce its own "feel-good" chemicals to induce a more positive state of mind. The antidepressants may be bicyclic (Prozac), or tricyclic (Elavil, Tofranil, etc.) – the drug of choice for many but one that causes major side effects (dry mouth, constipation, urinary retention) for some. If tricyclics cannot be tolerated, monoamine oxydase (MAO) inhibitors (Nardil or Parnate) can be substituted. MAO inhibitors cause severe headaches when taken with cheddar cheese, red wine, and a whole list of foods, beverages, and drugs. If you accept a prescription for an antidepressant, make sure that you understand the anticipated effects of the medication, as well as the restrictions and possible side effects. If you can't get the information from anyone else, discuss it with your pharmacist.

Remember that depressions are self-limiting. Even if you choose *not* to accept medication, the counseling offered by a therapist may help you sort out how much of the current situation is due to menopause and how much may be due to other events going on in your life. Much of the horror of depression is self-induced, because many women feel that they don't *deserve* to be depressed. Rather than acknowledge the depression and deal with it, they stumble along – for six months or a year – hoping that it will just go away. It will, but it may be beneficial to help it along a little!

Sexual Functioning

Because sexual function is linked to both physical and psychological states, it deserves a place of its own. It is often said that the important question involving sex at menopause is not *how often?* but *with whom?* There are many women alone during menopause (divorced, widowed, or never married). For too many, sexual activity becomes merely a decision about whether or not to masturbate.

For those women who *do* have partners, menopause may have a number of effects: intensity of both desire and response, increased desire but a slower response, infrequent or absence of desire with normal response when aroused, or decreased desire and response. From a psychological standpoint, such variation can be accounted for in a number of ways. One woman may experience the loss of reproductive ability as sexual freedom: desire and response may intensify. Another woman finds sexual activity enhanced by the risk of pregnancy: without the risk, desire wanes, although she may still respond. Still another woman has never enjoyed intercourse. Unless there is more time spent in undisturbed lovemaking or there are other positive changes (such as a new partner), both desire and response may disappear. It has been found that depressed women are more likely to dream about sex; like sex fantasies, sex dreams often translate into heightened desire. The possibilities are many.

> I have been separated for over four years (with no intimacy for years before that) and, in the intervening time, have married off three of the four children who had remained at home, had a hysterectomy, and a period of mild hot flashes. During a particularly stressful period, I had even developed what the doctor termed "senile vaginitis." What a dreadful term for a young lady of fifty-two! And then it happened – a "date" after thirty-five years. The friendship with this man, seven years my senior, turned into a full-blown romance and I couldn't believe my body's response! My hormones were dancing in double quick time and I don't remember anything as exciting as this even before age thirty-five. Here's to sex after fifty-three – it's wonderful!

Many women enter menopause with healthy levels of desire and response, but as they move into their fifties, they start to view *themselves* as less desirable. They find their bodies lacking – too fat, too flabby, too wrinkled; this may be a psychological concern, but it may also take into account a real change in physical appearance. Some women find that any kind of romantic caressing triggers a hot flash, and this alone can diminish one's response to a sexual overture. Some find that they are suddenly extraordinarily sensitive to touch; rather than "turning them on," it causes them to flinch. This is very difficult to explain to a partner. Women who once anticipated many orgasms now find that they are satisfied with fewer, perhaps one or two, and that the orgasms are not so intense as they once were.

> I am fifty-one and ended my periods two years ago, have had hot sweats for five years, but this is secondary to my real

problem, which began two years ago. For some reason, it seems that this, the most devastating problem of my menopause – the abrupt end of any sexual pleasure – has received very little print. Although I had read several books, for some time I did not realize that my problem was midlife-related. My innermost feeling is one of rage. I feel cheated and at times find it very difficult to deal with. I can now realize why marriages end. My own mate is also my best friend, so we are okay, but how I feel for women not so lucky!

Regular orgasm is known to be a precondition for a healthy vagina, and sexual activity (including masturbation) may help to prevent future problems, which, as already mentioned, include vaginal changes. The vagina tends to shorten and the walls grow thinner as menopause proceeds. Lubrication takes longer, requiring more foreplay. One menopause study tells us that one-quarter of menopausal women will experience discomfort during intercourse about 50 percent of the time. Sexual activity is more likely to remain pleasurable when the woman has a measure of control over the depth of penetration (as, for instance, lying on or beside her partner) and the confidence to voice her needs.

Sex after surgery

Women who have had surgery often have additional problems. Hysterectomized women may find that the quality of the orgasm changes, that the deep, inside-the-body feeling produced by a throbbing uterus is lamentably absent. Research suggests that orgasmic response may result from pressure-sensitive nerves in the cervix, which react to penile thrusting. In the absence of a cervix, the quality of the orgasm is bound to change. Many women who have lost a uterus and/or ovaries also report a complete absence of sexual arousal. Until recently, this was considered to be an individual and psychological response to surgery. Doctors assumed that women could enjoy sex only if they could make babies. It is now recognized that a fundamental physiological loss occurs in surgery, that the uterus itself may have important functions in *addition* to its acknowledged role as a "baby bag." It is important that women *know* that the amputation of sexual desire is neither intended nor foreseen. It is certainly not the woman's fault. This is just one more reason why hysterectomies and, above all, oophorectomies should be performed only after long and careful deliberation.

> I had a hysterectomy and partial oophorectomy at forty-three. The surgery left me a wreck. Although things were not great between my husband and me prior to the operation, the relationship took a nosedive largely because of my ensuing depression. I was teary and felt out of control. It took about a year for me to regain most of my former well-being. The biggest physical effect of the surgery has been the loss of desire for sex. Since my operation, my sex drive has lessened enormously. My husband and I are at a loss as to what to do.

If sexual function has been affected by surgery, there are avenues to be explored. If the problem is painful intercourse (dyspareunia), most doctors are very willing to provide a prescription for estrogen cream. When hormones are not advisable, water-based lubricating jellies or products such as Astroglide or Replens may make intercourse pleasurable once again. If the problem is absence of desire, your first step may be to establish credibility with your surgeon. For too many years, women have been told that absence of desire, or loss of libido, was an individual problem related to underlying feelings about sex *prior* to the operation. This is a no-win situation for a woman, because it is impossible to prove what one's "underlying" feelings are about *anything*, and it is hard to make a convincing case about how one used to feel or act in bed. (This is compellingly described in the provocative book *The Castrated Woman*, by Naomi Miller Stokes.)

Estrogen therapy rarely compensates for the loss of sexual desire, although it may make a woman feel better in other ways. ET tends to reduce the levels of circulating testosterone and, over time, may blunt the desire for sex. On the other hand, the administration of male hormones may restore some or all of the missing sexual desire, but to be effective, this may be have to be done within a short time of the surgery. The male hormone is variously described as an androgen or testosterone; testosterone is a form of androgen, a "male hormone," even though small amounts are produced in a normally functioning female – as is estrogen in a normally functioning male. Your gynecologist may be willing to read the relevant research and, if appropriate, prescribe for you. If the problem is the quality of the orgasm or the need for extended foreplay (to aid lubrication), then a sex therapist might be a valuable ally.

Sex during natural menopause

If sexual function is problematic during a natural menopause, it is more likely to be a temporary situation. The traditional explanation is that women are mourning the loss of reproductive ability and that this is unconsciously translated into a distaste for sex. Although this may be true for some women, it is certainly not true for the vast majority. More likely, the capacity for both desire and response will be affected by energy levels and feelings of self-esteem. Many women report an inability to experience intense feelings of sexual response. Those who are not fit may find that unusual exertion or orgasm may bring on a muscle spasm. Sexual difficulties arise in long-term relationships when we permit ourselves to draw invidious comparisons with "sex in the good old days," or when male partners – unwilling to admit that their own sex drive is not what it once was – blame lack of sexual activity on the women.

Women involved in *new* relationships report very few sexual problems during menopause; in fact, they often find that sex is better than ever. There are few studies of lesbian relationships during menopause, but those we have tell us that sexuality rarely deteriorates at this time of life, because nondemanding sex play is possible and mutually enjoyable. This suggests that strong bonds of affection and clear communication are crucial to mutually satisfactory sexual relationships during menopause. At one time, sexuality in the elderly was viewed as unnatural, even obscene. Today sexuality in the middle-aged is seen as merely the continuation of sexuality

CHAPTER 5

THE BIG
QUESTION:
HORMONES

As they approach menopause, many women worry about the hazards or benefits of estrogen therapy (ET) and combined hormone therapy (CHT), often without really understanding the issues. There is controversy about the benefits of hormones before, during, and after menopause. Yet only a fraction of the controversy reaches the popular press. This is partially because of the complexity of the situation and partially because of the enormous influence and power of the pharmaceutical companies and their views about what the public *needs* to know.

I was so appalled by the one-sided view of menopause presented at the 1991 meetings of the North American Menopause Society (that it is a deficiency syndrome requiring hormones for all or almost all women) that I put together a presentation – slides and commentary – to guide women through the steps of making a decision about hormone therapy. Many people have inquired about the availability of this presentation, some in the hope that it consisted of slides and a tape and could easily be shipped off. But the intricacies of estrogen therapy and new developments in the field make the decision-making process too complex to record permanently on tape. The situation is in flux and last-minute information must be accommodated. Therefore the presentation remains one to be made in person. It is with some trepidation that I attempt to summarize this updated version. Who knows what tomorrow may bring?

◆

We are in a unique situation on this continent: it is the only geographical area where gynecologists are so frequently used as primary-care physicians. In the countries of Western Europe, most women see a family physician (in some cases, *must* see a family physician) before they see a gynecologist. Gynecologists specialize in reproductive organs and are trained surgeons, whereas family physicians are more interested in other aspects of the patient's life and are more likely to consider other events or situations that might have an impact on her experience of menopause.

In North America, the pharmaceutical companies concentrate their sales efforts on gynecologists because these doctors write twice as many prescriptions for hormone therapy as do family physicians. (Also, hysterectomies are almost always performed by gynecologists, and women who have had hysterectomies use five times more hormone prescriptions than do naturally menopausal women.) Most doctors are too busy to research the claims and counterclaims of different drug manufacturers. They are influenced by the avalanche of publicity about hormones – advertisements in medical journals, reprints of research studies brought to their offices by pharmaceutical representatives – in addition to luncheons, dinners, conferences, and meetings sponsored, funded, or supported by drug companies.

To balance this one-sided view, many women and women's groups continue to publish articles, newsletters, and books stressing the other side of the story – potential side effects, the possibility of long-term adverse effects, and, most of all, the absence of properly designed studies of menopausal hormones.

The issues are complex, but even so, they are important concerns for women at midlife, and it is essential that women keep themselves informed.

What Hormones Are

Hormones are substances produced primarily by endocrine (ductless) glands, which means that the hormones are pumped directly into the bloodstream. Doctors who specialize in the study of hormones are called endocrinologists. They are the first to acknowledge that the glands of the female reproductive system operate in an intricate manner still only partially understood.

Major Glands and Reproductive Organs

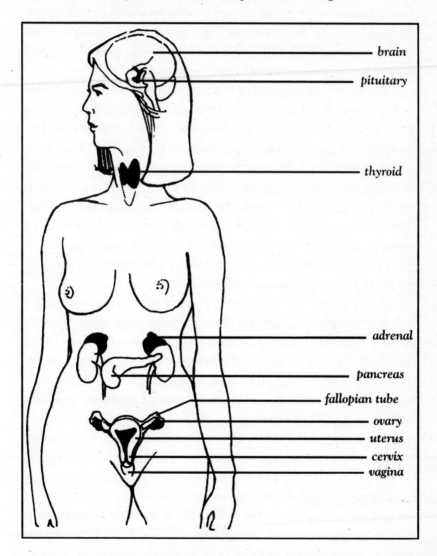

brain

pituitary

thyroid

adrenal

pancreas

fallopian tube

ovary

uterus

cervix

vagina

When we talk about estrogen produced inside the body (endogenous estrogen), we usually mean a particular kind of estrogen from the ovaries called estradiol. However, this is not the only form of estrogen in the body. Both the ovaries and the adrenal glands (perched on the kidneys) produce substances that are converted to another form of estrogen, estrone. Instrumental in creating strong bones, estrone is produced in very small amounts during the reproductive years but assumes more importance during menopause and postmenopause. A third kind of estrogen is also present – estriol, formed by the interaction of estradiol and estrone.

The process of estradiol production is initiated by the hypothalamus, a small gland in the brain. This gland, in turn, stimulates the nearby pituitary gland to produce FSH (follicle-stimulating hormone) and LH (luteinizing hormone), together known as gonadotropins. A follicle is the small vessel inside the ovary that contains an ovum, or egg. Stimulated by FSH, the follicle begins to produce estradiol, the major estrogen of the menstruating years. This hormone ensures a buildup of cells within the uterus (or womb) to provide a safe environment for a fertilized egg. A high level of estradiol in the blood signals the pituitary to decrease FSH production and to send out LH instead.

LH causes the follicle to burst, producing an egg; this process is called ovulation. The egg travels into the fallopian tube, while the spent follicle transforms itself into a corpus luteum (yellow body), which produces progesterone, the hormone that opposes or counteracts the effects of estrogen. Progesterone takes over during the latter part of the menstrual cycle (the days between ovulation and menstruation), and should the egg *not* be fertilized, progesterone ensures that the lining of the uterus (the endometrial tissue) is flushed out during menstruation.

Natural hormone changes at menopause
As one approaches menopause, the follicle may take longer to rupture, requiring more FSH, a higher level of estradiol in the bloodstream, and a thicker layer of cells inside the uterus. As a result, menstruation may be late and may result in a heavier-than-normal

Feedback System

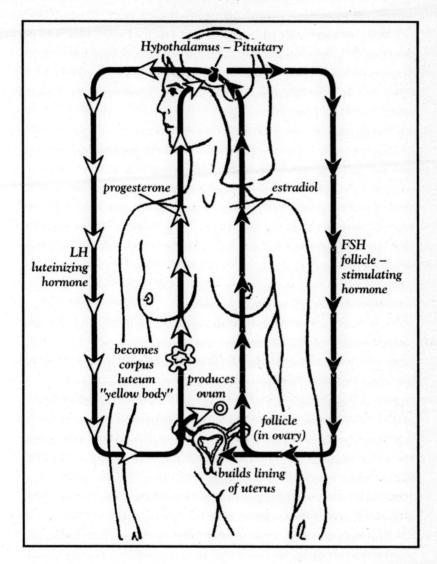

Hypothalamus – Pituitary

progesterone

estradiol

LH
*luteinizing
hormone*

FSH
*follicle –
stimulating
hormone*

*becomes
corpus
luteum
"yellow body"*

*produces
ovum*

*follicle
(in ovary)*

*builds lining
of uterus*

flow. A high level of FSH in the blood is one indication of menopausal onset and is one of the signs that doctors look for when doing hormonal assays to establish menopausal status. (Although the assay is most often part of a standard "one-shot" blood test, reliable results require a series of tests through one day and over a period of a month.)

By the time a hormonal assay confirms imminent menopause, most women are aware that a major change is under way.

Many women react to high levels of FSH by feeling blue and by temporarily losing interest in sex. This is characteristic not only of premenopause but also of the time just after childbirth, when high levels of FSH stimulate the first regular menstrual cycle after many months without periods.

It may take weeks, months, or years, but eventually the ovaries no longer produce eggs or follicles. Estradiol production declines, but the ovaries' production of both testosterone and the precursor to estrone increases with age. Because estrone is formed from substances produced by both the ovaries and the adrenals, and converted to estrone in the fatty tissue of the body, women with a little bit more padding on their bones tend to be more efficient at producing this form of estrogen.

Introduction of synthetic hormones

Estrogen and progesterone were first isolated in 1923, and the first synthetic forms of these hormones were made available in the 1930s. Immediately following World War II (1945 onward), there was a slow but steady increase in the numbers of prescriptions of estrogen as "replacement" therapy during menopause. Enormous strides were also made in the use and understanding of estrogen and progesterone in oral contraceptives. When the contraceptive pill was put on the market in the early 1960s, it was heralded as a historic breakthrough.*
Within a few years, estrogen therapy (ET) was similarly regarded. The 1960s were a decade of enormous faith in medical technology, and side effects or long-term effects were rarely considered.

The form of estrogen offered in ET was similar to that used in the contraceptive pill but at a fraction of the potency. This was a synthetic estrogen called ethinyl estradiol, which is still available in

---

* The formulation of this early pill delivered more hormones in a day than is contained in a month's supply of the new low-dose form. And today's pill still contains from three to five times more hormones than is prescribed in a standard dose of menopausal hormones.

some products. Another form of synthetic estrogen (diethylstilbe-strol, known as DES) was also strongly promoted as a way of mini-mizing the risk of miscarriage. No one knows how many thousands of women were given DES between 1941 and 1971.

We are still living with the fallout from the 1960s. There are many women who have been taking estrogen for decades and who are convinced that it prolonged their youth, reduced wrinkles, helped them stay slim, and postponed graying of their hair. In fact, all these claims for estrogen – once widely believed – have been found to be false.

After the initial infatuation with the pill, drawbacks became evident – including enormously increased risks of heart attack for women in their forties (most of them smokers). In response to con-cerns about these synthetic hormones, a new form of conjugated estrogen was developed, more nearly resembling human estrogen. This conjugated estrogen is estrone, rather than estradiol. Because it is collected from animals (Premarin, a trademark of Wyeth-Ayerst, is derived from *pregnant mares' urine*), it is often referred to as "natural" rather than "synthetic." This really means that the chemical composition of the estrogen more nearly corresponds to human estrogen.

Recent history of hormone use

From 1965 to 1975, menopausal estrogen was one of the four most commonly prescribed drugs in North America. But, in 1971, it was discovered that DES caused malformations and sometimes disease in the reproductive organs of the babies born to mothers who took DES. (It is now known that these children are six times more like-ly to be infertile and that the mothers themselves are also at sig-nificantly increased risk of breast cancer.) Following this tragic discovery, it was found that the rates of endometrial cancer for women taking menopausal estrogens was somewhere between six and fourteen times the norm, with the increase in risk depend-ent on duration and strength of the daily dose. Moreover, the increased risk remained for at least ten years after estrogen was discontinued.

The sales of estrogens plummeted after this revelation. At the same time, research projects multiplied in a frantic attempt to find ways to make estrogen more safe.

Estrogen, when not "opposed" by progesterone, as in the normal cycle (see page 80), stimulates the growth of cells in the uterus. When these cells are not washed away in a monthly menstrual period, the thickness and depth of the endometrium (lining of the uterus) can set the stage for a slow-growing cancer. Fortunately, it is a type of cancer that, if caught in time, is 97 percent curable – but at the price of a hysterectomy. (Therefore, taking estrogen without progestin, thereby incurring the risk of a hysterectomy, is not recommended. See chapter 7.)

A standard Pap test cannot detect endometrial cancer, so a woman who is on estrogen therapy and who has a uterus should have an endometrial biopsy every six months. This procedure is somewhat like a D&C. But instead of a curette, a cell sampler or a more recent innovation that uses a small-caliber, flexible plastic system is inserted through the cervix into the uterus. A sample of cells is then suctioned out for analysis. If the physician is experienced with this procedure, false negatives are substantially reduced. The newer suction curettes are more comfortable and avoid some of the pain involved in the use of standard cell samplers during the procedure and the severe cramping following it. (Women are told that the procedure is momentarily uncomfortable, but many women find the experience too painful to accept as a semiannual necessity.)

An alternative to endometrial biopsy is vaginal ultrasound, described on page 151. This is a painless way of monitoring endometrial health. Nonetheless, results of the PEPI (Postmenopausal Estrogen/ Progestin Interventions) trials show us that the risk of endometrial cancer, when using estrogen alone, increases to a point where estrogen alone, for the woman with a uterus, is to be strongly discouraged. Adding progestins or natural progesterone to the estrogen therapy is infinitely preferable.

How hormones are prescribed
For women with an intact uterus: For years, oral tablets have been the most commonly prescribed form of menopausal estrogen in

North America, and Premarin is the product that comes to mind when most physicians reach for their prescription pad. The Premarin tablet is available in four dosages – 0.3 mg, 0.625 mg, 0.9 mg, and 1.25 mg – of which 0.625 mg is by far the most common. Your prescription will also specify a progestin (often Provera) which, at 5 mg or 10 mg, is added to the estrogen during the last 10 to 14 days of the 28-day cycle.

This has been the most common regimen (method of administration) prescribed in Canada – that is, Premarin for days one through 25 of the month[*], with Provera added during the last 10 to 14 days of the cycle followed by a withdrawal bleed.

However, because of complaints about both the prolongation of periods and the side effects of Provera when this regimen is used, some women are taking progestins only every third month. An alternative is substituting a natural progesterone (i.e., Prometrium) for Provera to see if this can be better tolerated on a monthly basis. Why a progestin at all? Because it is important to shed the excess endometrial cells that have been stimulated by the use of estrogen.

But the Premarin/Provera cyclical combination is no longer the only game in town. As women hear about the benefits of natural, plant-based forms of estrogen (not to mention the hardships of the horses used to produce the urine), more prescriptions are being written for estrogen tablets such as Ogen or Estrace (see chart on pp. 87 ff.), for estrogen gel, or for one of the estrogen patches. Any of these estrogen products can be used in tandem with any progestational agent.

Synthetic progesterones (known as progestins or progestogens) are available in two basic types: one, medroxyprogesterone acetate (i.e., Provera) is progesterone-based; the other, the norethindrone type (i.e., Norlutate) is more androgenic, which means it affects the body as male hormones do. Both are synthetic progestins. Natural progesterone can be bought in the form of Prometrium, a product

---

* Day 1 of a menstrual cycle is counted from the day of the appearance of menstruation. In the absence of a menstrual cycle, day 1 is usually the first day of the calendar month. This is to make it easier for the woman and her doctor to remember. However, if the withdrawal bleed is inconvenient at the end of the month, day 1 can be arbitrarily fixed at any day of the month, provided this is consistent.

that rarely elicits the kind of side effects associated with synthetics, or in a prescribed and specially-compounded product containing powdered natural progesterone.

If you can't be bothered with two forms of medication, there is Premplus, a pill that combines estrogen and a progestin (medroxy-progesterone acetate). And there is Estracomb, a packet of patches that comprise an estrogen patch (changed twice weekly for two weeks) and a combination estrogen/progestin patch (also changed twice weekly for two weeks). See how easy they make it!

Another alternative – and becoming more popular every day – is to use both hormones on a continuous basis. This is the premise under-lying Premplus and Estracomb. The same effect could be achieved by using an estrogen patch (Climara, Estraderm, Oesclim, or Vivelle), or estrogen gel (Estrogel), or an oral estrogen tablet (Estrace, Ogen, or Premarin) coupled with a low-dose (2.5 mg) tablet of Provera daily or 100 mg of Prometrium daily. Ideally, this kind of regimen should elim-inate bleeding entirely (although there may be some breakthrough bleeding for the first few months), although it will not yield the bene-fits to blood fats that the cyclical regimen does (see page 95).

For women who have had a hysterectomy: If you are pre- or peri-menopausal and your ovaries have been removed, you may be given an injection soon after surgery, either Climacteron (an estradiol/testosterone combination) or Delestrogen (estradiol valer-ate) – a palliative to minimize the shock to your system due to the sudden loss of estradiol. Later, because there is no concern about endometrial stimulation (you no longer have a uterus), you can choose from the wide range of estrogen products listed above and shown in the chart. Be aware that some women react badly to one estrogen product but feel fine using another. So experiment.

You should also bear in mind that hysterectomy before normal menopause age is associated with increased risks of osteoporosis and heart disease. If you can use estrogen, you probably should. When you reach the age of 51 or 52 you may choose to discontinue it by tapering off very slowly. Your body will have become accustomed to high levels of estrogen and a sudden stop would be a shock. You can

Common Menopausal Medications

DRUG NAME & SOURCE	PRIMARY INGREDIENT(S)	SIZE	COLOR	DOSAGE/ USAGE	COMMENTS
BELLERGAL SPACETABS (tablets) Sandoz	Belladonna (anticholinergic) Ergotamine (antispasmodic) Phenobarbital (sedative)	One tablet contains: 0.2 mg belladonna 0.6 mg ergotamine 40 mg pheno-barbital	tricolor: green, orange and yellow	One tablet twice daily.	Contains lactose and tartrazine.
C.E.S. (tablets) ICN	Conjugated estrogens	0.3 mg 0.625 mg 0.9 mg 1.25 mg	green maroon pink yellow	One daily for 25 days (cyclic regimen) or one daily with progestins (continuous regimen).	Generic form of Premarin.
CLIMACTERON (injection) Sabex	Testosterone (androgen) and Estradiol	1 mL	liquid	Injected once every every 4 weeks.	Used primarily to treat women after removal of ovaries.
CLIMARA (patch) Berlex Canada	Estradiol	50–05 mg daily 100–.1 mg daily	translucent polyethylene film with an adhesive matrix	Applied twice weekly to abdomen or buttock. Not to be applied to breasts	A lower-dose patch (25) has been approved by the FDA for the U.S. market.
DELESTROGEN (injection) Squibb	Estradiol valerate	10 mg in 1 mL of solution	liquid	Administered in four 28-day cycles: Day 1, 2 mL injection (20 mg); Day 15, 250 mg of hydroxy-progesterone caproate + 5 mg of Delestrogen.	Prescribed infrequently.
ESTRACE (tablet) Roberts	Estradiol (derived from soy)	0.5 mg 1 mg 2 mg	white lavender turquoise	Initial dose is 1 or 2 mg daily; maintenance dose of 0.5 mg.	2 mg tablet contains tartrazine.
ESTRACOMB (patch) Novartis	Estradiol and Norethisterone (a progestin)	2 sizes: .05 mg estradiol daily OR estradiol + 0.25 progestins		Packet of 8. Following prescribed schedule, affix to abdomen or buttock. Change twice a week on same days.	Suitable for women with an intact uterus.

DRUG NAME & SOURCE	PRIMARY INGREDIENT(S)	SIZE	COLOR	DOSAGE/ USAGE	COMMENTS
ESTRADERM (patch) Novartis	Estradiol	.05 mg estradiol daily		Packet of 8. Affix to abdomen or buttock. Change twice a week on same days.	Suitable for women with no uterus.
ESTRING (vaginal ring) Pharmacia & Upjohn	Estradiol	Opaque ring		Insert deep into upper third of vagina. Delivers 7.5 mcg every 24 hours: lasts 3 months.	Should not interfere with sexual intercourse.
ESTROGEL (topical gel) Schering	Estradiol	Metered-dose pump 2 pumps = 2.5 g of gel.		Apply on hands and spread in thin, uniform layer on arms, abdomen or inner thighs.	Do not apply to face or breasts.
NORLUTATE (tablets) Parke-Davis	Norethindrone acetate (a progestin)	5 mg	salmon	2.5 mg–10 mg for 14 days of cycle	Contains lactose and tartrazine.
OESCLIM (patch) Fournier	Estradiol	25 – rectangular 50 – rectangular		delivers 25 mcg/day delivers 50 mcg/day	Self-adhesive polymer matrix backed onto a rectangular foam mounting with rounded corners.
OESTRILIN (vaginal cone) (vaginal cream) Desbergers	Estrone	cone: 25 mcg each; cream: 1 mg of estrone per gram of cream	cone: green, box of 10; cream: tube of 45 g with applicator		For treatment of dry vagina.
OGEN (tablet) Pharmacia & Upjohn	Estropipate (plant-based)	0.625 mg 1.25 mg 2.5 mg	yellow peach blue	One tablet daily	Contains lactose.

DRUG NAME & SOURCE	PRIMARY INGREDIENT(S)	SIZE	COLOR	DOSAGE/ USAGE	COMMENTS
PREMARIN (tablet) Wyeth-Ayerst	Conjugated equine estrogens	0.3 mg 0.625 mg 0.9 mg 1.25 mg	green maroon pink yellow	One daily for 25 days (cyclic regimen) or one daily with progestins (continuous regimen).	Contains lactose.
PREMARIN (vaginal cream) Wyeth-Ayerst	Conjugated equine estrogens	0.625 mg in 1 g of cream	white	Start with 1 mg daily and use more or less as vagina responds. Do not use before sexual intercourse.	Absorbed systemically. Severe cases may require 10 days of oral therapy.
PREMPLUS (tablets) Wyeth-Ayerst	Conjugated equine estrogens and medroxy-progesterone acetate	0.625 mg/2.5 mg 0.625 mg/5.0 mg	peach light blue	One daily (for women with intact uterus women only).	Lower dose prescribed to prevent osteoporosis. Higher dose for menopausal complaints.
PROMETRIUM (capsule) Schering	Natural progesterone (a progestin)	100 mg	round peach	2 capsules each evening for last 14 days of estrogen therapy, or 3 capsules (1 in a.m., 2 before bed) for last 14 days.	May be soporific. Progesterone is suspended in peanut oil.
PROVERA (tablet) Pharmacia & Upjohn	Medroxyprogesterone acetate (a progestin)	2.5 mg 5 mg 10 mg	orange blue white	5–10 mg daily for last 14 days of cycle or 2.5 mg daily on continuous regimen.	Contains lactose.
VIVELLE (patch) Novartis	Estradiol	37.5 mg/day 50 mg/day 75 mg/day 100 mg/day	Thin, circular, transparent patch	Affix to abdomen or buttock twice weekly Sold in packets of 8.	Less likely to cause skin irritation. Easy to clip to reduce dose when tapering off.

Notes: Tablets containing lactose may be difficult to digest. Tablets containing tartrazine may cause allergies in those sensitive to aspirin. Possible side effects of estrogen therapy include: swollen breasts (fullness at front rather than sides), burning when urinating or urge to urinate, premenstrual-like complaints, red flush or rash, increased facial or body hair, migraine, dizziness, headache, depression, changes in libido. Possible side effects of progestins include: swollen breasts (at the side, near armpits), backache, insomnia, dizziness, nervousness, somnolence.

minimize this by reducing the dose (halving tablets or taking them every second or third day), and gradually acclimatizing yourself to a normal postmenopause hormone milieu.

Spurred on by authors (e.g., by John Lee) whose books are widely available, the use of progesterone creams has become fashionable. Be aware, however, that over-the-counter creams containing substantial amounts of progesterone have been banned in Canada. There are a multitude of such creams available in the U.S.A. but there is no FDA regulation specifying the amount of progesterone contained. Assays done by Aeron LifeCycles of San Leandro, California, reveal that the creams – sold as containing "wild yam" or "discorea" or "natural progesterone" – may contain from 700 mg of progesterone to almost nothing or none at all.

ProGest, which is the best-known of the American creams, has a substantial amount of progesterone; preliminary studies have found that it can relieve hot flashes but has no effect on the development of osteoporosis, despite claims to the contrary. This is definitely a case of buyer beware.

It *is* possible to have a compounding pharmacy in Canada make up a cream, or other product, containing the exact amounts of estrogen, progesterone, or testosterone specified by your prescribing physician. You can find a pharmacy through the International Academy of Compounding Pharmacists at <www.iacprx.org>. Enter your postal code and you will be given a list of suitable pharmacies within a 50-mile radius. (There are also reputable compounding pharmacists who are not members of the IACP.) If you have a physician who is willing to work with you to find the precise formula to suit your biology, you are well on your way. If you don't know of such a physician, the pharmacist may have a suggestion.

(There are many alternative practitioners who believe that estriol, a milder form of estrogen, can be used without incurring any of the risk factors associated with estradiol – i.e., increased risk of breast cancer, gall bladder disease, etc. If you are contemplating having a cream compounded using estriol – perhaps on the advice of Wright & Morgenthaler – be advised that their claims for estriol have not been borne out in research. Estriol may incur the same kind of long-term risks as any other form of estrogen.)

For women who complain of dry vagina: The estrogen ring can be placed deep inside the vagina and can sit comfortably in place, dispensing small amounts of estrogen, for up to three months. Alternatives are the vaginal cones available from Desbergers or an estrogen cream which can be used lavishly to plump up the dry vaginal walls, and then used less frequently on a maintenance program. Again, if you have not had a hysterectomy, you should also use a progestin of some kind either for 14 days each month – or, with your doctor's approval, for 14 days each three months.

Once your vagina is friction-free, non-hormonal lubricants may be all you will need. You may also be surprised to know that regular sexual activity (intercourse and/or masturbation) is one of the best ways to maintain a state of comfort.

For women with depressed libido: A number of studies have found that healthy levels of sexual desire in women experiencing a natural menopause are *not* related to estrogen or androgen levels, but are more closely linked to a woman's overall state of well-being. Lack of sex drive in this kind of woman is often a temporary phenomenon (see pp. 75–76), and I would urge that other possibilities be considered and dealt with before resorting to treatment.

On the other hand, removal of the ovaries has been demonstrated to impinge on sexual desire, because the source of testosterone has been amputated. The good news is that, with the cooperation of a prescribing physician, it is possible to have a cream or jelly compounded at a pharmacy. As described by Dr. Susan Rako, this should contain a small amount of testosterone to smear on the clitoris. This may solve the problem of sexual arousal.

Who can or can't take hormones?

Estrogen and progestins, alone or separately, have profound effects on the body, and it is not clear exactly how progestins modify the effects of estrogen. High estrogen levels in the bloodstream have been associated with elevated blood pressure (hypertension) and blood clots (thromboembolisms or phlebitis), although the precise relationship is not clearly understood. Women who take oral estrogen are more than twice as likely to require gallstone surgery; creams and patches, however, don't carry this risk. Some of these negative effects have been traced to oral contraceptives that contain synthetic estrogens and, as mentioned earlier, at much higher doses than is normal for menopausal ET. But because it was not known whether the form of estrogen or the amount was the culprit, menopausal ET was, until recently, either not prescribed at all or prescribed reluctantly to menopausal women with a tendency to blood clots, gallbladder disease, or high blood pressure, *or* to women with a family or personal history of cancer. (Estrogen is known to stimulate certain types of breast tumors, primarily the estrogen-dependent type that occurs in younger premenopausal women.)

Uterine fibroids thrive in the presence of estrogen. Women with fibroids who experience pressure, pain, or heavy bleeding often notice a welcome relief of symptoms with the naturally occurring reduction of estrogen at menopause. Therefore, women with fibroids should avoid ET if at all possible.

> Much to my surprise, my doctor prescribed estrogen for depression. At the same time, he asked me if I knew that I had many large fibroids. I told him I *did* know and asked what their effect would be. He told me that they would cause erratic periods but made absolutely no mention of any other possible problems. Luckily, I had been on the ET for only six weeks before I read that estrogen would enlarge fibroids. I haven't taken estrogen since and find that exercise and vitamins keep the depression at bay as well as ET ever did.

Because obese women (women who are more than 20 percent over ideal weight) tend to produce a lot of estrone as a result of their large numbers of fat cells, those who are put on ET should be closely monitored.

Reasons for prescribing hormone therapy

Most women complain of some kinds of menopausal effects during the period of time when estradiol levels decline and estrone production increases (see page 82). Hot flashes are the most common complaint, and estrogen alleviates hot flashes for most women.

We still don't know exactly what causes a flash. A surge of LH has been noted to occur at the same time as a hot flash, but there is some other mechanism at work that hasn't yet been established. The flash may be caused by a *fall* in estrogen, suggesting that hot flashes may be due more to sudden changes in estrogen levels rather than, as commonly believed, the lack of estrogen. Adding estrogen from outside the body may alleviate hot flashes, but it may also postpone adjustment to new levels and new kinds of estrogen from inside the body.

When ET or CHT is prescribed to alleviate hot flashes, the usual recommendation is to take the lowest possible dose for the shortest possible time.

Estrogen is often prescribed to relieve depression, even though this is effective for only a small minority of women (see chapter 4). An interesting report from Britain notes that women on estrogen are more than twice as likely to commit suicide compared with those who don't use estrogen. This reflects the problem of inappropriate use of estrogen for women who are deeply depressed; hormone use does not solve the underlying problem. The stresses that contribute to depression are too often ignored.

> I am fifty years old and had a total hysterectomy at the age
> of thirty-three. Since then I've been taking ET and have now
> discovered that although the side effects are worsening,
> I am unable to get along without it. The most unusual of
> these side effects is a great sensation of heat on my left side.
> Besides this, my face and breasts swell, I'm continuously
> short of breath, and my legs ache. I attempted to go off estro-
> gen for a month, and although the side effects disappeared,
> I found myself getting terrible hot flashes and sinking into a
> terrible depression. I am now taking "nerve pills" prescribed
> by the doctor. Unfortunately, he has not been helpful in
> explaining how I could wean myself off the estrogen.

There is a very real concern that estrogen produces a psychological and physical dependency that some women find difficult to break. We hear from many women who are discontinuing use of hormones for a variety of reasons. Usually the doctor has recommended it but has not been very helpful about how to go about it. We counsel women to reduce the estrogen very slowly, either by obtaining a prescription for a lower dose or by cutting tablets into halves or quarters, or by taking the medication every second or third day so that the body can gradually adjust to lower levels. When using the Estraderm or Oesclim patches, cut a small part off, tape the edge, and use as usual. The Climara and Vivelle patches can be cut without taping edges. Any patch can be slowly reduced in size so that a steadily decreasing amount of estrogen is absorbed. Hot flashes may return for some time and may be very uncomfortable, but this is usually a temporary rebound effect. Eventually the body adjusts to the lower level of estrogen characteristic of postmenopause.

Although estrogen causes the skin to retain more moisture, and the slight swelling sometimes makes fine wrinkles less visible, estrogen does not prevent wrinkles. For women with very fine, transparent skin, estrogen helps maintain a cushion of collagen under the outer layer of skin, adding a degree of firmness.

Estrogen may also relieve cystitis (the sensation of burning during urination) and other complaints of the vaginal/urinary system, including dry vagina. (See chapter 2 for more about estrogen cream.)

Estrogen is often prescribed for women who experience a loss of sex drive after reproductive surgery. Sometimes this is helpful because it compensates for the sudden loss of vaginal lubrication during sexual arousal; it may also help restore sensitivity to the nipples. But women who have experienced oophorectomy lose the minute amounts of testosterone that contribute not only to libido (the desire for sex), but that appear also to influence a global sense of well-being. For these women, the addition of testosterone may make a big difference. The problem is that testosterone is difficult to control: even in slight overdoses, it can cause acne, an enlarged clitoris, a more masculine voice, or unwanted body hair – and may very well contribute to an increased risk of heart disease and breast cancer.

Since 1985, both ET and CHT have been widely promoted as ways to prevent both osteoporosis and cardiovascular disease. In both cases the hormone therapy is prolonged, and serious questions arise about the advisability of putting *most* women on hormone therapy in order to protect only those at risk. More information about osteo-porosis and cardiovascular disease is available in chapter 6. Here we will examine the benefits and drawbacks of using hormones.

Exactly how estrogen functions to halt the loss of bone that cul-minates in osteoporosis is not completely understood, although it is known that estrogen stimulates the release of calcitonin, a hormone from the thyroid gland. Calcitonin, in turn, stops the release of bone tissue into the bloodstream. We know that women who have had a number of pregnancies (during which estrogen levels soar) are less vulnerable to osteoporosis, as are women who are overweight. (Some of this may be due to the benefits of the extra weight putting stress on bone; some may result from the higher production of estrone.) On the other hand, women who have their ovaries removed begin to experience bone loss immediately after surgery, and this bone loss proceeds more swiftly than in normally menopausal women (see chapter 6).

There is no doubt that estrogen is a valuable medication for women at risk. There is also no doubt that the numbers of women at risk are enormously inflated as a result of the vast numbers of hys-terectomies, and particularly oophorectomies, that are performed on this continent. Healthy ovaries are routinely and unnecessarily removed from women over forty, or over forty-five – putting them at enormously increased risk for osteoporosis *and* cardiovascular disease.

A year and a half ago, I had a hysterectomy and oophorec-tomy. I was started on estrogen and progesterone and had bowel failure. The estrogen was taken away and my bowels started to function. The gynecologist I was seeing gave me hormone injections (estrogen plus testosterone) and another kind of synthetic estrogen over the course of about five months. I was then sent to an endocrinologist about the thirty-five pounds I had gained. His advice was to take a tranquilizer and stop worrying.

I went back to my family doctor really upset. I thought I was going off the deep end. I was having severe hot flashes, feeling depressed, suffering from severe anxiety, and had lost

almost all interest in sex. He sent me to another endocrinologist, who did a complete workup and found elevated
levels of testosterone. He put me back on estrogen tablets,
which did not help.

Lately, I've stopped taking the estrogen and progesterone.
My body is now readjusting and finally I feel in control of
myself and of my body.

✦

Estrogen supplementation has been strongly promoted as a form of
protection against cardiovascular disease, largely based on its ability
to increase blood levels of high-density lipoproteins (HDLS) by 10 to
15 percent. (The importance of this is explained in the next chapter.) This presumed benefit was reinforced some years ago on the
basis of results from the ongoing Nurses Health Study.

This study involved 122,000 married female registered nurses in
the U.S. who were between thirty and fifty-five when the study
began in 1976. These nurses have been followed at two-year inter-
vals since and, in 1991, it was found that, based on ten years of data
on 48,470 postmenopausal women, those taking estrogen were found
to be at significantly decreased risk for major coronary disease.

This was a major factor in the decision to promote estrogen as a
way of protecting women from heart disease, but these results have
been called into question by newer studies. Before we even get to the
studies, however, it is worth mentioning that 27,000 North
American women participating in the hormone replacement arm of
the massive Women's Health Trial were notified, in the spring of
2000, that more women on ET or CHT were suffering heart attacks,
strokes, and blood clots than the controls (that is, women not taking hormones of any kind). These events were noted in a very small
number of women, not enough to halt this arm of the trial, but it was
a surprising and sobering development.

During that same year (2000), a study of women with established
cardiovascular disease (average age of 65) found that, over a three-
year period, the women did *not* benefit from being on either Premarin,
or the usual Premarin/Provera regimen. This news came two years

after HERS (the Heart and Estrogen/progestin Replacement Study) was published, reporting that, in year one of the study, women on CHT had more coronary events than women *not* on hormones, including three times the number of blood clots.

Because the Women's Health Trial has a few years yet to run, the implications of these findings are still somewhat uncertain. Although estrogen is capable of raising the level of HDLS in the blood, there is something else going on that appears to offset this potentially protective function *in some women*.

At first it was thought that the added progestins were diluting the benefits – but that no longer seems to be the case. Some physicians believe that the negative effects on risks of heart disease show up only during the first year of treatment and that, after the first year, estrogen is beneficial. But if you are among the 1 percent of women who suffers a heart attack, stroke, or potentially fatal blood clot as a result of hormone therapy, the first year of treatment is a year too long!

Potential side effects of ET and CHT

One of the major concerns with both ET and CHT is noncompliance – that is, women who receive a prescription and never have it filled, or they have it filled but then stop taking the pills (or using the patch) as they wish. One study of 301 women who had been prescribed hormones noted that only 30 percent ever took the medication. Noncompliance is a major problem in evaluating the effectiveness of ET and/or CHT, but it is an aspect of hormone use that is consistently ignored.

Linked to this problem of noncompliance is the issue of side effects. Hormones are powerful medications, and in the drive to produce standardized dosages, the very individual reactions of many women are ignored or discounted. Estrogen therapy alone can cause increased appetite; bloat; headaches; swollen, tender breasts; nausea; vomiting; cramps; dizziness; fluid retention; rashes; visual disturbances; depression; or changes in levels of sexual desire (libido). Some of these side effects can be eliminated by adjusting (usually reducing) the dose, but some cannot. Estrogen may also cause breakthrough bleeding, which means bleeding between the expected times of menstrual bleeds.

Progestins (alone or in CHT) can cause swollen breasts, water reten-tion, headaches, decreased sex drive, fatigue, and increased appetite.

Moreover, there is considerable evidence that ET, used for five years or more, contributes to an increased risk of breast cancer. Preliminary data suggest that this risk is increased with the addition of progestins (i.e., CHT), but this has yet to be confirmed.

The relationship between estrogen use and breast cancer is still under discussion. There have been over forty studies; some have found no relationship but a substantial number (including the respected Nurses Health Study) have found significant increases in cases of breast cancer after some years of use. These findings are triv-ialized by many gynecologists because of studies that have found *no* increased risk. My view is that, until it has been established that estrogen cannot stimulate potential cancers, we should pay attention to *any* well-constructed study that finds an increased risk. A few years ago, it was generally thought that use of estrogen for ten years or less would not increase the risk of breast cancer. Newer studies suggest that the 'ten years or less' would be more accurately estimat-ed as "five years or more."

How to Make a Decision

The continuing controversy over risks and benefits of estrogen (ET) and estrogen-plus-progesterone (CHT) makes it difficult (but not impossible) for the individual woman to make an informed choice.

If menopause is viewed as a deficiency disease or condition, as it is by some medical practitioners, then it follows that some kind of treatment will be viewed as beneficial to *all* women approaching menopause. If menopause is seen as a natural stage of biological devel-opment, however, estrogen will be seen as medication useful for those most seriously affected (that is, those who have had an artificial menopause, those at serious risk of cardiovascular disease or osteo-porosis, and those few women who suffer an intolerable menopause).

Some people feel that drugs were invented to cushion us from discomfort and stress, and that to spurn such relief is silly. Others believe that we swallow too many drugs without thinking of the consequences, and that sound nutrition and other changes in daily routine should be adopted before resorting to drugs. These differing attitudes influence many decisions about ET.

ET or CHT should be prescribed for a woman only after she has had a thorough medical examination, including not only blood pressure, a pelvic exam, and a Pap smear, but also measurement of blood lipids, a breast examination and mammogram, and, ideally, a bone-density scan. Her doctor will usually insist on a checkup in three months, and every six months thereafter. This means that women on ET or CHT are *more* likely to have regular medical checkups than women not receiving estrogen. Because of this consistent surveillance, including endometrial biopsies, Pap tests, and breast exams, if these women *do* develop signs of a disease, it is more likely to be caught early.

Thus if a woman no longer has functioning ovaries, and particularly if the loss of ovaries occurs before the normal age of menopause, ET is probably a sound decision. If loss of sex drive results from oophorectomy, ET with added testosterone may be the only effective therapy. When the ovaries are removed, the uterus is usually removed as well: where there is no uterus, there is no worry about endometrial cancer. Given the enormously increased risk of osteoporosis to women who go through early menopause as a result of surgery, ET is probably a wise move. (It is also worth noting that oophorectomy significantly reduces the risk of breast cancer.)

Similarly, because any form of premature menopause increases the risk of osteoporosis and perhaps of cardiovascular disease as well, women who go through an early menopause for any reason should seriously consider ET or CHT.

On the other hand, we have little to no information about the protective effects of a healthy life-style – regular vigorous exercise, no smoking, little or no alcohol, a low-fat, high-fiber diet. It is quite possible that these pluses more than make up for the loss of ovaries. We just don't know.

Women who go through natural menopause but who find hot flashes, night sweats, or associated discomforts absolutely intolerable may choose to take CHT. This is a quality-of-life choice and it should be respected. There is no evidence that taking CHT for a period of less than *five* years increases the risk of breast cancer. Some women find that a short course of ET or CHT allows them to overcome the fatigue and emotional stress that makes decision-making impossible. Once they are back on their feet, they can decide whether to continue with hormone therapy or to make other changes in their lives that may help them withstand the stresses of menopause. I've heard from women in high-powered jobs or in the public eye who have chosen to take hormones in their fifties in order to minimize the discomforts of menopause, but who intend to wean themselves off the medication very slowly in the privacy of their well-deserved retirement years.

> There is no official standard or protocol for administering
> or prescribing CHT. Furthermore, no conclusive studies
> have been performed that indicate which regimen is most
> beneficial, and there have been no studies that meet design,
> duration, and sample size requirements for determining
> conclusively the risks and benefits of long-term use of
> CHT. (OTA, *The Menopause, Hormone Therapy and Women's
> Health*, 69:1992)

Fortunately, women at particular risk for osteoporosis now have options other than hormone therapy. Two non-hormonal products, Fosamax (alendronate) and Didrocal (etidronate), are approved for both the prevention and treatment of osteoporosis; others (risedronate and pamidronate) are approved for treatment only. An anti-estrogen, raloxifene (Evista), is also approved for prevention of osteoporosis. All three are prescription products.

Although there has been a flurry of interest in ipriflavone, an over-the-counter dietary supplement composed of a synthetic version of isoflavones and rumored to be bone-building, a randomized, controlled test of this substance has found that it does not build bone, does not prevent bone loss and that, on the contrary, it con-tributes to a reduction in white blood cell count (lymphocytes).

The Osteoporosis Risk Profile (next chapter) is a rough guide to bone loss but this should be verified by a bone scan. If results indicate minimal bone loss, regular vigorous exercise may avert the need for medication. If you prefer, for whatever reason, not to take estrogen, there are alternatives. The important thing is not to be coerced into anything, but to make the decision from a position of informed choice.

The newest rationale for ET – to minimize the risk of cardiovascular disease – complicates matters even more. Although it is true that women are much more likely to die of heart disease than of breast cancer (currently 30 percent of women die of some form of CVD, compared with 4 percent of women who die of breast cancer), the advantages of ET are just not that clear-cut.

There is no question that "natural" estrogens in oral tablets maintain or increase blood levels of HDLs (the "good" lipids in the blood), but they also increase triglyceride levels. Many studies have found that high levels of total cholesterol and of the "bad" LDLs substantially increase the risks of heart attack, but *only when triglyceride levels were also high*. It is suspected that triglycerides make the blood more likely to clot, which starts most heart attacks. It may well be that not only low HDLs and high LDLs contribute to increased CVD risk, but that high triglycerides are an important and neglected part of the equation. (See also chapters 6 and 8.)

Women who have a family history of heart attack or stroke, or who suffer from chronic high levels of cholesterol (hypercholesterolemia) may decide to take their doctor's recommendation and use ET in the hope that theory will translate into practice and validate their choice. However, given the uneven performance of estrogen therapy in combatting coronary disease, more cardiologists are prescribing statins – Zocor (simvastatin), Mevacor (luvastatin), Pravachol (pravastatin), etc., to lower cholesterol levels – rather than sending their middle-aged female patients back to a gynecologist for an estrogen prescription. There is growing evidence that cholesterol levels mean less and less as a predictor of heart disease as a woman ages. Many healthy women recognize that there are other preventive strategies to reduce the risks of CVD and actually find the prospect of heart disease less frightening than the prospect of breast cancer. After all, we have to die of *something*. What if we manage to avoid heart disease, then develop breast cancer at age eighty?

The whole question of estrogen use is highly complex, and there are no simple answers. Given the long latency period of breast cancer, it is hard to know just what was happening in a woman's body fifteen or twenty years ago that has resulted in a diagnosis of cancer today. Because types and doses of hormones have changed so much over the past few decades, it is impossible to go back and trace their possible effects. But even when we *do* have more definitive information, the decision about whether to seek or to accept hormone therapy has to be an individual one, based on the quality of life of one individual woman and taking into account the many unknowns that still plague us.

CHAPTER 6

INCREASED HEALTH RISKS AT MENOPAUSE:

OSTEOPOROSIS, HEART DISEASE, BREAST CANCER

For many of us, menopause comes as a shock. We are forced to become aware of what we take for granted – our bodies and our health. Because our bodies no longer respond, perform, acquiesce in the ways they once did, we are forced to recognize our age and our mortality. Although some women find this difficult to accept, it does have its compensations.

Menopause reminds us to take stock of our health and to initiate steps to withstand the threats to good health that increase with age. It gives us the chance to decide whether we will be easy targets for the diseases of old age or if we are willing to make an effort to stay healthy – not only for our own benefit, but for the benefit of those who would have to take care of us.

The word *osteoporosis*, which means porous bone, was first named by a German pathologist in 1930. Although extensive studies were done on postmenopausal osteoporosis throughout the 1940s and 1950s, it did not reach the popular press or stir public concern until the 1980s. Osteoporosis is not a disease; it is the end result of many processes that lead to a state where bone mass is less than the needs of body mass. Bone may appear normal, but on close inspection it is found to be riddled with holes, somewhat like a dry sponge.

The bones of the forearm (near the wrist) and the thigh (at the hip) may become dangerously fragile, whereas bones in the spine threaten to collapse from the effort of holding up the body.

Heart-related medical conditions – hardening of the arteries, high blood pressure, heart disease, or stroke account for more than half the disabling health problems on this continent. Before age sixty, twice as many men are affected; after age sixty, women are as vulnerable as men. Menopause does not, of course, *cause* heart disease, but after age fifty-five, women are more likely to have high blood pressure (hypertension) than men. Any book about menopause must include the bad news: menopause brings with it the increased risk of heart disease, particularly for those who experience surgical menopause. Once a woman has had one heart attack, her chances of experiencing a second are greater than a man's. And women are less likely to survive heart surgery.

We may be only vaguely aware of the heightened risks of osteoporosis and of cardiovascular disease, but many of us know, in some small, secret place, that we are also moving into a high-risk category for breast cancer. In fact, 65 percent of new cases of breast cancer occur in women over fifty.

Osteoporosis

Bone is both the vital framework of the body and a storehouse for calcium and other minerals. Bone cells are constantly being formed, used, and sloughed off, much like the outer layer of skin is cast off. The outer layer of bone sheds cells into the bloodstream, and the cells are excreted. Most of the calcium in the body exists as bone or teeth, but there is a constant circulation of calcium in the bloodstream. It is the balance between the loss of bone cells (resorption) and the formation of new cells (absorption) that determines bone density and presumed durability of bone.

During the growing years – until the mid-thirties – the absorption of calcium into bone exceeds the resorption of calcium into the bloodstream, so bones get bigger and stronger. Although we inherit a tendency to strong or weak bones, the density of bone can also be affected by the amount of calcium in the diet and by the weight and activity of muscle pulling against it – the action involved in all movement. If there is a family tendency to dense, durable bone, and if this is complemented by good nutrition and exercise habits, a negative balance (that is, losing bone faster than it is formed) can be tolerated for some years. Men are generally heavier and more muscular than women, and until very recently, this difference was accentuated by the wider participation of men in sports. This is the major reason that most men in our society do not show evidence of osteoporosis until well into old age. Because the life expectancy of the male is considerably less than that of the female, the problem of osteoporosis is overwhelmingly a woman's health problem in this society. (Although there have been slight changes, the average life expectancy of a woman is about six or seven years more than that of a man.)

There are two different kinds of osteoporosis: primary and secondary. Primary osteoporosis develops as a consequence of natural aging *in both men and women.* Secondary osteoporosis simply means that the condition is brought on, or worsened, as a result of other problems – prolonged bed rest, glandular disorders (hypoglycemia, hypothyroidism, Cushing's syndrome, Addison's disease, or diabetes mellitus), bone marrow tumors, kidney dialysis, and/or as a side effect of medication. Some of these medications are oral corticosteroids (e.g., prednisone for asthma), anticonvulsants (Dilantin), diuretics containing furosemide, or antacid preparations containing aluminum. Prolonged use of thyroid medication (particularly if the dosage is not reduced appropriately as a woman ages) increases the likelihood of osteoporosis, as does use of psychotropic drugs (tranquilizers, antidepressants, or sleeping pills).

Whether primary or secondary, the osteoporotic woman is at risk for crush fractures of the lower and/or upper back (the latter is more evident as "dowager's hump"), for wrist fractures ("old lady's" or Colles' fracture), and for hip fractures – not at menopause but later in life. The immobility and complications resulting from hip fractures are responsible for the deaths of 20 percent of older women, usually within four months of the accident.

Osteoporosis is more common in affluent, northern countries, where bone density peaks in the fourth decade of life. Most women then start losing between .02 percent and .07 percent of bone each year. During the two to five years immediately following the last menstrual period, bone loss may accelerate to as much as 2 percent as a result of lowered estrogen levels, after which bone loss slows to the rate more characteristic of premenopause.

Women who have had multiple pregnancies, who eat red meat infrequently, who do strenuous labor, and who are overweight (by Canadian standards) are not likely to develop osteoporosis. These are the characteristics of the majority of women throughout the world. Moreover, black women rarely suffer from osteoporosis because they inherit denser bones than do whites. Asians in America, however, are vulnerable, presumably because they tend to be small boned and slim and because they do not inherit a dense bone structure. (Ironically, Asians in China and Japan appear to be not as susceptible to osteoporosis. We are not sure why.)

Surgical removal of the ovaries doubles the risk of osteoporosis. Because North America leads the world in the number of hysterectomies performed, and since many surgeons still routinely remove ovaries from any woman over the age of forty or forty-five, the high incidence of osteoporosis is probably due to unnecessary elective surgeries. Interestingly, this is not viewed as a problem in the medical literature!

In addition to accelerated bone loss as a result of gynecological surgery or as a side effect of certain medications, some women fit into the category of "fast loser." Not a great deal is known about why certain women are "fast losers," but a urine test known as Osteomark is now being used, in conjunction with other testing, to identify women at risk. (The test measures compounds that are present in urine in direct proportion to the amount of bone collagen resorbed.)

Estimates about the prevalence of osteoporosis vary enormously. It is commonly believed that one in four women going through natural menopause, and one in three women experiencing surgical menopause, will be at serious risk, but this risk may only arise if and when a woman reaches her ninetieth year. Moreover, estimates of risk do not discriminate between those affected by less serious consequences of osteoporosis (minor vertebral compression, forearm fractures) and those disabled by crush or hip fractures or their aftermath.

The Osteoporosis Risk Profile (shown here) will give you an idea of your individual risk factors. Use this profile to help decide if you should be taking steps to protect yourself.

The best way to prevent osteoporosis is to have strong bones. Heredity is one factor, but women with strong bones will have consumed lots of calcium (milk, cheese, dark-green vegetables) during their early adult years and engaged in regular exercise that puts stress on the bones. Because bone is built as the result of the mechanical pull of the muscles, exercises that involve use of the whole body are best – walking, running, rope jumping, and racquet sports. At one time it was thought that swimming was not particularly beneficial for osteoporosis because of water's buoyancy. Now it has been found that swimming does help, although it cannot offer the same degree of needed stress to the bone that weight-bearing exercise does. Weight or resistance training is good for the bones. Bicycle riding will help the bones of the lower body, but may not strengthen the bones of the arms and shoulders. (A cyclist who plays the piano regularly may have an advantage!)

Diagnosis
Bone loss is intensified by consuming too much caffeine (in coffee or tea) in place of calcium-rich milk, by high consumption of phosphorus (in red meat and some cola drinks), by smoking, and by not doing regular weight-bearing exercise. In addition to calcium, your diet should also include adequate amounts of Vitamin D ("the sunshine vitamin"), and three minerals: magnesium, manganese, and boron.

Women with fair, transparent skin seem more vulnerable to osteoporosis; the decline in mineralized collagen (bone) is reflected in the absence of opaque collagen under the surface of the skin. This skin type is also characteristic of rheumatoid arthritis sufferers, but what link exists between this and osteoporosis is not yet established. (Osteoarthritis, a noninflammatory degenerative joint disease, seems to add to the risk of osteoporosis. Women who have had a hysterectomy are at greater risk for both osteoarthritis and osteoporosis.)

The Osteoporosis Risk Profile[*]
By Diane Palmason

This chart is intended to help you assess the extent to which you are at risk for spontaneous fractures of the spine, hip, and wrist that occur in persons with postmenopausal osteoporosis. Listed below are a number of factors that affect your risk profile, including those that you can affect through your lifestyle ("takens"), as well as those that are genetically determined ("givens"). Beside each factor find the statement that best applies to you, note the number beside that statement, and write the number down in the right-hand column.[**]

GIVENS   **SCORE**

Age:

Female–under 35 1	35–50 3	51–65 7	Over 65 12	____
Male–under 50...............1	51–65 2	66–80 3	Over 80 4	____

Heritage:

Black 1	Oriental..............1	Mediterranean Middle Eastern...3	Nordic Anglo-Saxon......5	____

Complexion:

Dark 1	Ruddy/Olive.......2	Fair/Pale 5	____

Heredity:

No known bone problems in family.......................1	Relative over 60 with bone disease 3	Parent with bone disease 4	Relative under 60 with bone disease 5	____

Wrist Size:

Over 6 ¼" 1	6" to 6 ¼"" 2	5 ¾" to 6"...........3	under 5 ¾" 4	____

Height:

over 5'8"........................1	5'5" to 5'8" 2	5'2" to 5'5" 3	under 5'2"...........4	____

Body Type:

Mesomorphic (high muscle, low fat)..........................1	Endomorphic (high fat, low muscle)..............6	Ectomorphic (low fat, low muscle)..............6	____

Gynecological Status:

Still menstruating or postmenopausal after 50..........................1	Menopausal or postmenopausal 46–50 3	Early menopausal 45 or under........5	Surgically menopaused before 45 7	____

TOTAL OF GIVENS: ____

[*] Originally appeared in *Fitness Leader*, October 1984 issue. Reprinted by permission.

[**] Deduct 5 points if estrogen replacement therapy was started within one year after surgery or early menopause, 3 points if started more than three years after surgery or early menopause.

Strategies and Remedies

TAKENS   SCORE

Exercise:

| Total body exercise 4 or more times weekly ....0 | Total body exercise 1 to 3 times weekly.......3 | Total body exercise at least 3 times monthly....6 | Avoid physical activity............12 | ____ |

Eating Habits:

a) Calcium Intake***

| 4 or more servings of low-fat dairy products daily.................0 | More than 2 servings of dairy products daily.....3 | 2 or fewer servings of dairy products daily.....6 | Avoid dairy products ....12 | ____ |

b) Protein Intake

| Avoid red meat altogether.......................0 | Seafood and white meat of poultry only........1 | Meat 3 times weekly or less ....3 | Meat 4 times weekly or more.............. 6 | ____ |

Drinking Habits:

a) Caffeine Intake

| Avoid caffeine and tannin beverages.......................0 | Decaffeinated drinks and/or tea only ....2 | 3 or fewer cups of coffee/ tea daily..............3 | 4 or more cups of coffee daily....................6 | ____ |

b) Alcohol Intake

| Weekly average fewer than 2 beers or 8 oz. wine or 3 oz. spirits ....0 | Weekly average 2–4 beers or 8–16 oz. wine or 3–6 oz. spirits .....2 | Daily average up to 2 beers or 8 oz. wine or 3 oz. spirits ....4 | Daily average more than 4 beers, 16 oz. wine or 6 oz. spirits ....8 | ____ |

Tobacco Use:

| Non-user ....0 | Occasional cigarette only, fewer than 14 weekly ....2 | Daily smoker, fewer than 10 daily ....5 | 10 cigarettes daily or more ....8 | ____ |

TOTAL OF TAKENS: ____

ADD GIVENS FROM PREVIOUS PAGE: ____

FINAL TOTAL: ____

Assess your risk according to the following: 8 to 25 – risk well below average; 26 to 48 – risk below average; 49 to 59 – risk generally average; 60 to 82 – moderate risk; 83 to 100 – considerable risk. Note that this chart is not intended to diagnose whether you are, or will be, osteoporotic. It is simply an indication of the extent to which you are similar to women who have been found to have osteoporosis. For an accurate diagnosis, it is necessary to have a bone scan.

*** Subtract 3 points if you take a daily calcium supplement that provides from 500 to 1500 mg of calcium.

Periodontal disease, which involves changes in the bones that hold the teeth in place or in the gum surrounding that bone, *may* be a sign of osteoporosis. One clue may be greater loss of bone in the upper jaw, which contains more trabecular bone than the lower. (Cortical bone, which constitutes 80 percent of bone mass, is the hard and shiny kind that makes up the outer surface. The inner part is called *trabecular*, or *cancellous*, and this more porous type of bone is characteristic of the major portion of the vertebrae. Trabecular bone is more vulnerable to osteoporosis than is cortical bone.)

Since the calcium that circulates in the blood helps to monitor muscle contraction, one early indication of osteoporosis may be knotting of the large muscles, particularly in the calf. (Low levels of potassium may also cause this kind of cramping, which can often be relieved simply by adding potassium-rich foods, such as bananas, to the diet.)

Seventeen years ago, I had my uterus and ovaries removed. I was taking estrogen for six years after that but finally decided to give it up, as I dislike the idea of long-term dependency on a drug. Lately, I've been experiencing unbearable muscle spasms in my legs. I started eating a banana a day in order to alleviate the cramps, with absolutely no results. My doctor is as stumped about this as I am. Even regular exercise has not helped.

A common symptom of more advanced osteoporosis (usually postmenopausal) is lower back pain, either as muscle spasm or dull ache. If the pain persists for several weeks and then disappears, it may signal the crushing of a vertebra. When bones are fragile, the smallest exertion – a sneeze or a hug – can cause a fracture.

Loss of height, particularly in the upper body, may also be an indication of osteoporosis. Some loss of height occurs naturally as one ages – caused primarily by the contraction of the hip-flexor muscles. But measurements of upper-torso size may be an indication of bone health.

Although all the methods used to diagnose osteoporosis are non-invasive, painless, and involve little discomfort, some are more effective than others. Routine X-rays show bone loss only when 20 to 30 percent of bone is affected, often too late to take preventive action. CAT scans (computerized axial tomography) are available in large medical centers but must be specifically adapted and made available for osteoporosis. This often occurs only when the condition is so advanced that confirmation of a diagnosis is sought.

To have a CAT scan, the woman is placed on a cot that is slid into a metal cylinder. The body is bombarded with rays that provide a computer printout of bone density. The CAT scan, neutron activation analysis (which is even rarer), and absorptiometry all use radioactive materials, but expose the patient to only a fraction of those used in standard X-rays.

DEXA (dual energy X-ray absorptiometry) machines are the gold standard for bone density tests. They measure bone mass in the spine and arm – using very low levels of radiation – then calculate and display results on a computer screen. Dual photon absorptiometers (DPAs) and single photon absorptiometers (SPAs) are older versions of this technology and are considered less reliable. The SPA measures forearm bone only.

Ultrasound has a number of theoretical advantages in measuring both bone quantity *and* quality, takes only three to five minutes, and is rapidly becoming available. It involves immersion of the heel bone in a circulating water bath with the results displayed on a computer screen as with the DEXA machine. Density of heel bone has been found to correlate nicely with the health of other bones in the body.

More and more hospitals are making bone scans available to the general public, so your physician may be able to make arrangements for a bone scan if you are worried about the risk of osteoporosis. The printout generated by a scan will tell you the state of your bones relative to other women your age. If your bone density is in the adequate range, you may decide to continue exercising regularly, while taking calcium and Vitamin D. (In areas of the country that get little winter sun, Vitamin D is important. Spinal bone mass can be improved by taking 500 IUs of Vitamin D daily.) If the bone mass is "borderline," you may wish to have another scan in twelve months. If the results put you into or near the "fracture zone," you may decide either to take estrogen or to take a non-hormonal medication. Estrogen halts bone loss whereas other medications can rebuild lost bone.

The most telling symptom of osteoporosis is, of course, the broken bone. Once one fracture occurs, there is a tendency for other bones to break: 95 percent of osteoporotic women have at least five more fractures in the ten years following the first.

Nonprescription remedies

There is a great deal of controversy over the role of calcium, particularly calcium supplements, in the prevention of osteoporosis among women who are premenopausal (still menstruating regularly), perimenopausal (having erratic or skipped periods), or postmenopausal (whose last period occurred at least twelve months earlier). Because calcium is a nutrient, not a drug, its effects are not immediately apparent. And calcium alone is *not* enough to reverse the bone loss that marks the five years following the last menstrual period. But its effectiveness in building bone during the premenopause and in strengthening bone in the years following year five of postmenopause have been convincingly documented.

Most women consume only about 500 to 600 mg of calcium in their daily diet, which is below the RNI (recommended nutrient intake) of 800 mg daily for women between fifty and seventy-four, weighing 63 kg (138 lbs.). And the RNI itself is probably inadequate. According to a consensus panel of the National Institutes of Health in the United States, women *not* on estrogen should aim for 1400 to 1500 mg daily; those on estrogen need about 1100 mg.

Dietary sources of calcium are shown on page 114. To consume enough calcium daily, a woman must diligently drink a quart of skim milk, or maintain a high intake of canned salmon or sardines (including bones), plus green, leafy vegetables. If this is impossible on a regular basis, it may be advisable to include a calcium supplement.

Calcium supplements may offer inadequate protection for women at *high risk for* osteoporosis. But calcium supplements, *in combination with regular exercise*, are helpful for the average woman.

These supplements are available in many forms: the most common are calcium carbonate, calcium gluconate, calcium lactate, calcium citrate and dibasic calcium phosphate. If you read the labels, you will find that calcium carbonate is 40 percent elemental calcium, dibasic calcium phosphate is 31 percent, calcium citrate is 21 percent, while lactate contains only 13 percent elemental calcium, and calcium gluconate only 10 percent. *It is the amount of elemental calcium that is crucial.*

In other words, a 600-mg tablet of calcium carbonate provides 240 mg of calcium, whereas the same size tablet of calcium lactate provides only 79 mg of calcium. Calcium gluconate provides even less. The labels of any calcium product should indicate just how much elemental calcium you are getting. If you divide the price of the bottle by the units of elemental calcium, you will have a guide to the cost of that particular supplement. What you are looking for is the most economical product to do the job.

Cheaper isn't always better, however. To make sure your calcium tablet will be properly absorbed, put it in 200 ml (6 oz.) of white vinegar and see how long it takes to dissolve. If it is still virtually in one piece after thirty minutes, it is not likely to be effectively absorbed in the stomach.

Some forms of calcium are tolerated better than others. Calcium is absorbed more effectively along with a dairy product (milk or yogurt) and, for maximum benefit, just before bedtime. More new bone tissue is laid down while you sleep. If you have a bad reaction – indigestion, bloat, flatulence, constipation – to a particular calcium supplement, don't give up on calcium entirely. Try another product until you find one that you can tolerate. Avoid products that include other nutrients, such as Vitamin A or Vitamin D. When evaluating a product, it's better to deal with one nutrient at a time.

Calcium supplementation without exercise is probably a waste of money, because the calcium is likely to be excreted. Again, exercise is the key to prevention:

Table of Calcium-Rich Foods

Amount	Food	Calcium
	DAIRY PRODUCTS	
	Cheese	
1 oz.	Cheddar Cheese	204 mg
1 oz.	Colby	194 mg
1 cup	Creamed Cottage	126 mg
1 cup	Dry Curd Cottage	46 mg
1 cup	2% Cottage	155 mg
1 cup	1% Cottage	138 mg
1 oz.	Cream Cheese	23 mg
1 oz.	Feta	140 mg
1 oz.	Gouda	198 mg
1 oz.	Monterey Jack	212 mg
1 oz.	Mozzarella	147 mg
1 oz.	Part-skim Mozzarella	183 mg
1 oz.	Low Moisture Part-skim Mozzarella	207 mg
1 oz.	Provolone	214 mg

Amount	Food	Calcium
1/2 cup	Ricotta	257 mg
1/2 cup	Part-skim Ricotta	336 mg
1 oz.	Swiss	272 mg
1 oz.	American Processed	174 mg
	Milk	
1 cup	Whole Milk	291 mg
1 cup	Low-fat Milk 2%	297 mg
1 cup	Low-fat Milk 1%	300 mg
1 cup	Skim Milk	302 mg
1 cup	Goat's Milk	345 mg
	Other	
1/2 cup	Ice Cream	90 mg
1/2 cup	Ice Milk	115 mg
1 cup	Plain Yogurt	274 mg
1 cup	Plain Low-fat Yogurt	415 mg
	SEAFOOD	
1 cup	Oysters	226 mg

Amount	Food	Calcium
7.5 oz.	Pink Salmon	160 mg
3.75 oz.	Sardines	240 mg
1 cup	Shrimp	147 mg
	VEGETABLES	
1 cup	Bok Choy	116 mg
1 cup	Broccoli	140 mg
1 cup	Collards	357 mg
1 cup	Dandelion Greens	147 mg
1 cup	Kale	206 mg
1 cup	Mustard Greens	193 mg
1 cup	Turnip Greens	267 mg
	OTHER	
4 tbsp.	Almonds	85 mg
2 tbsp.	Blackstrap Molasses	280 mg
4 tbsp.	Tahini	270 mg
3.5 oz.	Tofu	128 mg

Research on postmenopausal women comparing exercisers to sedentary controls have consistently found exercise to be beneficial to bone health as measured by calcium balance, bone mineral content and cortical diameter. Particularly encouraging is that exercise has been found not only to prevent bone loss, but actually to increase bone mass. In Smith's study of women aged sixty-nine to ninety-five, sedentary controls lost an average of 3.29 percent of bone mineral over thirty-six months, while those in an exercise program increased bone mineral by 2.29 percent. (Gannon, p. 118)

You will need adequate Vitamin D to use the calcium properly. If you don't get regular exposure to sunlight (fifteen minutes a day is all it takes) and don't drink milk (which has 100 IUs of Vitamin D in each cup), you may need supplements: 400 to 800 IUs daily.

Magnesium, manganese, and boron are minerals that are also necessary to maintain bone strength. The RNI for magnesium is 210 mg, easily available from whole-grain breads and cereals, and fresh green leafy vegetables. Studies have suggested that low levels of manganese in the diet are related to poor calcium absorption and that the diets of most menopausal women are chronically short of manganese. There are no RNIs established for manganese or boron, but 2 to 5 mg of manganese daily is considered adequate; this is available from whole grains, nuts, fruits, and vegetables. Preliminary studies suggest that boron may be vital to bone health, partly by influencing estrogen levels during postmenopause. A diet that includes lots of noncitrus fruits (apples, pears, cherries, grapes), green vegetables (cabbage, broccoli, beet greens), nuts, and legumes (dried peas and beans, lentils) will provide the necessary 2 to 6 mg.

Prescription remedies

If your physical makeup and family history strongly predispose you to osteoporosis or if you have had a bone scan and are perilously near the "fracture zone," you may want to consider taking estrogen to halt further bone loss. Estrogen halts loss of bone (although you must *continue* to take estrogen to enjoy this benefit). The most common dosage to prevent bone loss is one 0.625 mg tablet of Premarin daily, although an estrogen patch at 50 mcg offers equivalent protection. There is also evidence that a reduced dose of Premarin (0.3 mg) *with daily exercise* may be as effective as 0.625 mg. Note, however, that estrogen cannot build new bone in the absence of exercise.

Once a woman is five years postmenopausal, the period of greatest bone loss is past. This is valuable information, because estrogen is often prescribed as if it worked equally well for all women and as if all women were equally in need of it.

Etidronate disodium (Didronel) has been available for some years as a treatment for Paget's disease. Now, repackaged with calcium carbonate under the name Didrocal, it is being used to treat osteoporosis. The tablets (400 mg) are taken daily for 14 days, followed by calcium carbonate (500 mg of elemental calcium) for 76 days, in a 90-day cycle. Another bisphosphonate, alendronate (Fosamax), has also been approved for ingestion morning and night. Didrocal is less expensive than Fosamax but provokes more side effects. Other bisphosphonates – risedronate (Actonel) and pamidronate (Aredia) – are also available for treatment of severe osteoporosis and may one day also be approved for prevention of bone loss.

Calcitonin treatment, like estrogen, merely halts bone loss. In North America, it has traditionally been administered by injection and is not only costly but often involves unpleasant side effects. After some years of use in European countries and the U.S.A., calcitonin as a nasal spray was approved for use in Canada. This product, Miacalcin, is packaged in a spray bottle containing 14 metered doses of 200 IU of calcitonin, to be used once a day in alternating nostrils. The manufacturers recommend that it be used in conjunction with 1000 mg daily of calcium enriched with vitamin D.

Another possibility is raloxifene (Evista), a SERM – or selective estrogen receptor modulator – a sort of "designer" estrogen. These products are like the older forms of synthetic estrogen in some ways but not like them in others. Raloxifene was approved for the prevention of osteoporosis in 1998 and is being strongly promoted by its manufacturer on the grounds that it does not increase risks of uterine cancer. (This is to differentiate it from another SERM, tamoxifen, that is used to reduce the risk of breast cancer recurrence, but which increases risks of both uterine cancer and blood clots. Raloxifene is being tested against tamoxifen to establish which is the better preventative for breast cancer and with what side effects.) It is really too soon to tell if raloxifene will live up to its publicity.

And that's not all. Progesterone therapy (usually consisting of Provera) has been used to strengthen bone in women who cannot take ET. Progesterone appears to be most effective in building trabecular bone (which makes up most of the vertebrae) and it is hoped that these benefits will also accrue to those who choose natural progesterones. No reliable data on this yet.

I am 66 years old and have been suffering from osteoporosis for two years. Last winter, I broke my hip in a fall and have since been extremely conscious of my calcium and Vitamin D intake. My doctor seems to feel, however, that if I begin to take estrogen now, the osteoporosis will decrease. Is this true?

Estrogen *halts* bone loss, but estrogen with calcium, magnesium, vitamin D, and – most important – exercise, can *rebuild* lost bone. So can calcium plus supplements and exercise, but not to the same degree.

At the present time, women approaching or experiencing menopause hear mostly about estrogen as the way to prevent osteoporosis. Experts are now seriously considering starting estrogen, as a preventative to osteoporosis, when a woman is in her later years – late 60's or 70's. This might protect women when they really need it, without involving an unnecessarily increased risk of breast cancer due to long years of estrogen use.

The fear of osteoporosis is based on projections of the costs of caring for old women with broken hips. These projections are based on our current situation – an aging population that has never been encouraged to eat bone-building foods or to exercise regularly. Since most doctors have been trained to look for medical solutions to problems presented by their patients, since menopause has been only fleetingly mentioned in medical school, and since hormone medications have been publicized so widely, most do not think of adjustments in diet, or changes in exercise patterns, as solutions. Younger women who are more aware of the risks of osteoporosis – and of heart disease – are more likely to get regular exercise and more likely to benefit from remedies which may be less expensive and less risky.

Heart Health

Until recently, most studies dealing with heart disease focused on men. What was generally accepted to be true (in terms of vulnerability to cardiovascular disease, or CVD) was based on information about males. For instance, Type A personalities – tense, ambitious overachievers – are considered more prone to CVD. More often than not, this means male, middle-class management types. Among women, however, those earning low wages, whose jobs are low in status, are at greatest risk. These women are more likely to have blue-collar jobs and to be working class.

Moreover, doctors are more likely to dismiss complaints of chest pain from women, judging it to be an emotional rather than a physical symptom. Men are also much more likely to be scheduled for angiography, a procedure involving injection of a dye that allows the blood vessels in the heart to be viewed on X-rays. And women who have bypass operations are less likely to survive, probably because, by the time their complaints are taken seriously, they tend to be both older and more seriously ill than male patients. The susceptibility of women to cardiovascular disease and the quality of medical treatment given to them are undergoing new and very welcome scrutiny. We have a lot to learn.

◆

The cardiovascular system is made up of four basic components: (1) the pump (or heart); (2) the pipes (the veins and arteries); (3) the control system (the nerves that cause the heart to beat, valves that ensure the one-way flow of blood, etc.); and (4) the material moving through the system (the blood). Problems may be caused by: (a) clogging of the pump or pipes; (b) leaking or bursting of the pump or pipes; (c) breakdown in the control system; or (d) changes in the blood as it moves through the system. Some problems result from a single cause, but most arise from a combination. The major culprit is the clogging of the pump or pipes.

The clogging starts when elements carried along in the blood invade, coat, then accumulate on the inside of a blood vessel. The composition of the blood may be partly to blame, or the inner lining of the arteries may be roughened with wear, so that it catches filaments as they flow by. But the particular pattern of the clogging and the locations are highly individual, and no one knows what causes a particular pattern. As the passage for the blood narrows, the heart must work harder to pump the blood into all the tissues. As the artery walls lose elasticity, they may weaken and balloon out. This is called an aneurysm. Should the aneurysm leak or burst, the consequences can be deadly.

In other cases, thrombi (blood clots) may hinder blood flow to the brain (cerebral thrombosis) or to the heart (coronary thrombosis). If the thrombus is swept along to another site to block circulation of the blood, it is an embolism. A pulmonary embolism is in the lungs, a cerebral embolism occurs in the brain.

When artery walls thicken and lose flexibility, the condition is known as arteriosclerosis. When the clogging is caused by deposits of certain kinds of fat (atheromas), the condition is known as atherosclerosis. In order to force blood past these obstructions in the arteries, the heart must work harder, which causes the pressure of the blood in the arteries to rise. This results in high blood pressure or hypertension.

Hypertension

A blood-pressure reading is a routine part of every medical checkup. Blood pressure is charted according to the force of the heart pumping (the systole) over the force of the heart at rest (the diastole). Although the reading varies, depending on amount of physical exertion, time of day, and emotional state, a consistent and acceptable reading is anything between 100 and 135 for the first number and between 50 and 85 for the second. A reading of 140 over 90 (written as 140/90) is considered borderline. The lower figure seems to be more important when predicting trouble.

Some women react to estrogen therapy with a sudden increase in blood pressure, which is why doctors recommend that women on estrogens have their blood pressure checked every six months.

Hypertension is known as the silent killer because you may have it and never know it. A person with high blood pressure is three times more likely to have a heart attack, eight times more likely to have a stroke, and five times more likely to experience heart failure. Hypertension may also lead to eye problems or kidney failure.

It was once thought that blood pressure naturally got higher as one aged. Now it is known that blood pressure can be kept at a healthy level through diet, exercise, reduced salt intake, not smoking, careful weight watching, and adequate calcium intake.

I am a woman of fifty-three who has been experiencing menopausal problems for five years. I was always a workaholic, smoked a lot, and generally ignored my health. I refused to let menopause slow me down, although my blood pressure was high and I suffered from insomnia. Two years ago, I had a heart attack. I've now changed my life-style completely: I've stopped smoking, I eat better, and exercise regularly. My blood pressure is back to normal – thank God! – and I feel one hundred percent better.

When blood pressure rises, a doctor has the option of prescribing medication (usually a diuretic) or enlisting a patient's cooperation to change bad habits. Diuretics promote the excretion of fluids and salt, but the use of diuretics also causes frequent urination and loss of vital potassium. Strict antihypertensive drugs (and there are many of these) often involve even more side effects. One widely used drug, reserpine, has been found to increase the risk of breast cancer; other drugs lead to restless sleep and frequent awakenings. In addition, the benefits of hypertensive medication can be canceled by the interactive effects of other medications – oral contraceptives, appetite depressants, or nonsteroidal anti-inflammatory drugs (NSAIDs) prescribed for arthritis.

More and more doctors recognize that a nondrug approach to controlling blood pressure may be as effective as medication, or more so. As much as one-third of the population is known to be sodium sensitive; for these people, a sharp reduction in salt intake may stabilize borderline blood pressure, which may then be treated with commonsense precautions – no smoking, more exercise, and a healthier diet.

Stroke

Leaking or clogging in the brain can lead to a major stroke (cerebrovascular accident, or CVA). Or, if the leaking is intermittent and minor, a transient ischemic attack (TIA) can result. Ischemic simply means that the tissues are being starved of oxygen. If blood cannot reach brain cells, the starved cells will die. And although some experts suspect that brain cells *may* have the capacity to regenerate, they don't know how to promote this regeneration. The damaged cells may never be reactivated. If many cells are affected, the result may be paralysis, loss of speech, or other deficits, depending on the part of the brain affected. Recovery is slow because new nerve pathways must be forged and old skills painfully relearned. If only a few brain cells are affected, the effects are more subtle – tingling in the extremities, momentary dizziness or weakness, etc. TIAs may be shrugged off as temporary inconveniences, but the cumulative effect of a series may be loss of brain function, even senility. After a series of transient ischemic attacks, the patient's behavior may be similar to that of a person suffering from Alzheimer's disease.

Heart attack

If leaking or clogging occurs in the coronary arteries, the diagnosis is coronary heart disease (CHD) or ischemic heart disease (IHD). The pain resulting from the heart's loss of its own blood supply is called angina pectoris. The usual progression is atherosclerosis of the coronary arteries, followed by ischemic heart disease (which makes itself known by the pain of angina), and finally a heart attack. The section of the heart fed by the clogged artery cannot function for more than five minutes without an adequate blood supply. When heart muscle is damaged, myocardial infarction occurs.

There are, of course, many other problems resulting from the leaking, clogging, and bursting of the heart and blood vessels. Some conditions are the result of birth defects; some result from scarring caused by a disease such as rheumatic fever; some are caused by bacterial infection or by conditions that affect specific parts of the heart or arteries.

Arrhythmia

Any disturbance to the natural rhythm of the heartbeat is arrhythmia, which is caused by a malfunction of the control system. The natural pacemaker of the heart functions inside the atrium, or upper chamber of the heart, and governs the regularity of the beat. Tachycardia is a condition in which the heart begins to beat too fast (at about 180 beats per minute). If the heart speeds up even more, it may flutter at around 250 beats per minute, or flatten out completely during fibrillation.

A less dramatic but more common complaint during menopause is paroxysmal atrial tachycardia which does *not* lead to flutter or fibrillation and may occur in otherwise normal, healthy persons. Occasionally it may be caused by migraine activity (see chapter 2). Tachycardia is very different from the more common palpitations, which is merely an unpleasant awareness of the heart beating and is often felt at times of anxiety or panic.

If you experience episodes of tachycardia, you should be referred to a cardiologist to rule out rapid heart rate caused by the lower chamber of the heart, which is a more serious condition.

Medication is often routinely administered to alleviate arrhythmia, but studies indicate that skipped beats or a temporarily "racing heart" rarely have anything to do with heart disease. In fact, some studies suggest that medication may cause more problems and that most people with heartbeat irregularities can expect to live as long and as healthily as anyone else.

The valves of the heart, arteries, and veins are a major part of the cardiovascular control system because they ensure that the blood moves in the desired direction. Malfunction of the heart valves is not uncommon. When the mitral valve doesn't close properly after each beat, this can be heard through the stethoscope. In fact, prolapse of the mitral valve (Barlow's syndrome) is said to affect 15 percent of women over the age of thirty. Echocardiography (a painless procedure that bounces sound waves into the chest cavity) can confirm the diagnosis with relatively little risk. With mitral valve prolapse there may be minor chest pain, some palpitations, and some shortness of breath after exertion. The greatest concern about the condition is the risk of heart infection, which can follow from standard dental procedures. Women with mitral valve prolapse are advised to keep a prescription for antibiotics on hand and to start ten days of treatment prior to any dental work (including teeth cleaning).

> For the past year, I have suffered from severe heart palpitations and a very fast heartbeat. Cardiologists cannot find anything apart from a prolapse of the mitral valve, which apparently is of no concern. I'm sure I have a spine full of arthritis, which causes pains in my neck, shoulders, and arms, and which some days is just about more than I can bear. This all hit me within a year after a lifetime of being just fine. I'm only forty-three and when I mention to doctors that perhaps I could be starting my change of life, they laugh at me. They think I'm too young for that. I get dizzy spells and tire very easily. I have had all the tests to be had and everything appears normal. I'm on beta blockers to slow my heart down and I have side effects from this medication. So right now I feel like I have nowhere to turn. I know that I'm feeling like hell, but the doctors apparently cannot or will not do anything for me.

Varicose veins

The venous valves, particularly those below the waist, are responsible for varicose veins, which may occur quite aside from any conditions affecting the arteries. One can have varicose veins without any worry about arteriosclerosis or clogged arteries. Varicose veins are estimated to affect at least 20 percent of women and perhaps 8 percent of men, and they seem to run in families. They may show up as a visible network of enlarged veins in the legs, as a painful ache from the veins deep inside the legs, or as hemorrhoids. They may be aggravated by pregnancy, when veins swell to accommodate the enormous increase in circulating blood.

Although varicose veins are not attractive, they are rarely life threatening. Superficial veins may require elastic stockings (either heavy-duty elastic or the less noticeable support hose). These should be put on first thing in the morning before getting out of bed. Restrictive garments – girdles, knee-high stockings, tight shoes, or boots – and long periods of sitting or standing (especially if one is overweight) will make varicose veins worse. When sitting, the legs should be elevated as much as possible. A diet high in fiber and in Vitamin C has been found to be beneficial. The superficial spider-web-type marks that often accompany varicose veins may be treated with injections of saline solution, which often causes them to disappear. Ask your family physician for the name of a varicose-vein specialist or sclerotherapist. Relatively painless surgery is required to "strip" bulging surface veins, so that the blood is forced to circulate through deeper veins. The major risk with varicose veins is the possibility of blood clots (thrombi) or phlebitis, inflammation in the deeper veins.

Phlebitis

Although thrombophlebitis also involves veins, it is more serious and indicates the presence of both blood clots and inflammation. The presence of varicose veins increases the risk of phlebitis, as does taking the contraceptive pill. Deep-vein phlebitis is more difficult to treat. The inflammation (which causes a dull ache and/or swelling) may signal the presence of a clot (thrombus), which must be dissolved using anticoagulants. This produces severe side effects in about 5 percent of patients. If the clot is not dissolved, it may loosen and move through the system to become a life-threatening embolism. Symptoms of an embolism include chest pains or shortness of breath.

Blood clots may form after a blow to the legs, or a fall, or when blood flow is slowed down because of immobility during illness or after surgery. Phlebitis is not common and is frequently misdiagnosed, but newer diagnostic tools (such as impedance plethysmography) are increasing medical expertise. Women prone to phlebitis are advised to exercise regularly and to give up smoking. Bedridden patients should be carefully monitored, and where necessary, low-dose anticoagulants should be used to increase blood flow.

Risk Factors for Cardiovascular Disease

Most of the factors that lead to increased risk of CVD can be controlled. The exceptions are heredity and age/sex. Let's deal with these first.

Heredity
Certain individuals may inherit a tendency to blood-chemistry conditions that put a strain on the heart, such as high cholesterol levels or a prolonged, abnormally high white-blood-cell count. Black women have higher rates of both heart disease and hypertension than whites, despite the fact that their blood-cholesterol levels are often lower. The tendency to obesity, to dark hair in and around the inner ear, or to a crease across the earlobe are also inherited, and each indicates an increased risk for CVD. And varicose veins may pose a minor risk. On the other hand, some of us also inherit a tendency to high HDL (high density lipoprotein) levels, which serve to protect against heart disease. With some detective work, most of us can discover our inherited tendencies and work to offset them.

Age/sex
Age increases the risks for all forms of cardiovascular diseases; moreover, *women who experience any kind of menopause before the age of forty-five – forty in particular – are at greater risk.* Women generally

enjoy greater protection from most cardiovascular problems (compared with men) until the late fifties, but are more prone to hypertension. Although it has been assumed that high levels of estrogen provide the extra margin of protection to premenopausal women, ET administered to men results in more heart attacks. It is possible that high levels of testosterone in the male make him vulnerable, and that the risk diminishes as testosterone levels fall with age.

Diet

A high-fat diet significantly increases the risks for CVD, and excessive salt consumption is a primary factor in hypertension. There is still disagreement about the possible effects of coffee, although filtered coffee is safer than boiled or percolated (unfiltered) coffee.

Cholesterol is an animal fat found in many kinds of food (oils, meats, and eggs) but it is also manufactured in our bodies. The human liver can produce all the cholesterol we need. Because cholesterol and other fats (called triglycerides) are not water soluble, they must be bound to other molecules that act as carriers in order to circulate in the blood. The carrier molecules are called lipoproteins. Lipoproteins fit into four groups according to density. Low-density lipoproteins (LDLs), in combination with cholesterol, are responsible for the congestion of artery linings and are a potential cause of heart disease. They are the "bad" lipids. High triglyceride levels may also be dangerous for women over age fifty. High-density lipoproteins (HDLs), on the other hand, pick up stray bits of cholesterol and dispose of them, counteracting the dangerous effects of the LDL/cholesterol combination. They are the "good" lipids. Menstruating women tend to have higher levels of HDLs than do men, which is one reason that younger women enjoy prolonged protection from cardiovascular disease. The concern with diet is to extend this protection past the menopausal years, so that women will remain at a lower risk for heart disease as they age.

A more complete explanation of the function of lipoproteins and how to evaluate cholesterol and lipid levels can be found in chapter 8. However, most of what we know about the role of the various kinds of lipoproteins in relation to heart disease has been the result of large-scale studies done on men, who benefit from both the lowering of LDLs and the raising of HDLs. The blood chemistry of women is different. For them it is the shift in HDLs that is crucial.

The most recent theory suggests that excess iron in the system can be correlated with the probability of heart attack. The argument is that menstruating women are not prone to heart disease because the monthly bleed excretes excess iron, which can be stored indefinitely in the body. Further research is required, but it's possible that iron-rich foods (such as organ meats and spinach) may be poor choices after menopause.

Alcohol
Low alcohol consumption is related to a lower probability of heart disease, hypertension, osteoporosis, and breast cancer.

Smoking
Inhaled nicotine constricts the peripheral blood vessels, increasing resistance and thus blood pressure. A smoker is six times more likely to develop hypertension. Nicotine interferes with the liver's ability to dispose of blood fats, allowing more cholesterol and triglycerides to circulate and to clog up the system. At the same time, carbon monoxide in the cigarette smoke permits cholesterol to invade the artery lining and acts to reduce the oxygen-carrying capacity of the red blood cells. The risk of heart attack is directly related to the number of cigarettes smoked. Women who smoke are advised not to take the oral contraceptive pill after the age of forty (even with the newer low-dose pills) until more consistent data are available.

Stress
Risk of heart disease is also affected by stress. There is "good stress" and "bad stress." Stress produces a rush of epinephrine (another word for adrenaline) – a chemical that increases heart rate, blood pressure, and blood flow to the extremities. Evolution has programmed us to react swiftly to stress with heightened alertness and unusual physical strength. This enables us to run from the threat that produced the stress. We experience "good stress" when we rise to the occasion in

a well-matched game of tennis or flog ourselves to swim another ten laps. However, if the chemicals are not dissipated through physical exertion, they can have damaging effects on the body. If these stressful episodes occur too frequently, or if any part of the cardiovascular system is weakened or damaged, chronic hypertension may result.

Stress occurring in a situation of powerlessness may be even more harmful. There is an enormous difference between the stress generated by high-powered women who thrive in pressure-cooker situations and the stress endured by those women exploited by others, whether in a dead-end job or a no-win relationship. It is women in the latter situations who run the greater risk of hypertension and heart disease.

Weight

A weight gain of 20 to 25 percent over ideal weight is considered obesity and poses a significant risk. Women who are overweight appear to be at greater risk for CVD than are overweight men, particularly if the extra weight is carried on the abdomen. If the waistline disappears and a "pot" develops, this is a warning sign. How the weight is distributed may be more important than sheer poundage. A gain of 10 to 15 percent over ideal weight (which may protect against osteoporosis and hot flashes) may be acceptable, provided the difference between waist and hip measurements remains roughly the same (e.g., instead of 66 cm [26 in.]/91 cm [36 in.] a change to 76 cm [30 in.]/101 cm [40 in.]).

Exercise

One of the best predictors of heart disease is a sedentary life-style. During exercise, most of the energy requirements for the muscles are provided by the blood. In order to supply increased oxygen during exercise, more blood pounds through the system as the heart rate speeds up, the rate of perspiration increases, and a larger amount of oxygen is extracted from the bloodstream by the organs and tissues. If the activity level is maintained, the arteries open up to increase the blood flow to working muscles. Exercise thus promotes the elasticity of the arteries, enhances blood flow, raises the level of HDLs in the blood, and reduces the probability of substantial weight gain. Regular aerobic exercise that sustains the heart rate at an optimum level for at least twenty minutes is one of the best ways to prevent cardiovascular problems. Chapter 8 provides a way of figuring out for yourself if you are getting sufficient, regular aerobic activity.

Diabetes

Women with diabetes are six times more likely to develop heart disease, compared with male diabetics, who incur double the risk.

◆

We are handicapped by the limited information available about heart disease in *women* (as opposed to heart disease in men). Yet there appear to be significant differences not only in the development and symptoms of some kinds of cardiovascular disease, but also in the effects of certain treatments. Some women continue to produce ovarian hormones for many years after the last menstrual period; it is not known what effect this has on the risks of heart disease. Nor do we know what, if any, relationship exists between women who experience migraine, or severe varicose veins, or intense hot flashes, or palpitations associated with menopause. The relentless promotion of ET to protect women against CVD has obscured the fact that while ET enhances blood lipid profiles, it may act in other ways that are harmful. Moreover, some studies have demonstrated that cholesterol levels are not always predictive of heart disease, particularly as a woman ages. We need more information about women's individual risks.

Nevertheless, some women know they are at increased risk for CVD. Women who are dealing with known risk factors should be anxious to see the results of the Women's Health Initiative, a large-scale trial that may establish definitively whether ET is protective in the long term. In the meantime, they may want to use their cardiologist's non-hormonal medications, just to be on the safe side.

Even though we have known for some time that women who undergo artificial menopause continue to experience higher-than-normal risks of heart disease, there is no evidence of any concerted effort by the medical profession to reduce the unacceptably high rates of elective hysterectomies and oophorectomies. Until we have more accurate information, we are again faced with a situation where millions of women may be induced to take estrogen unnecessarily. This might be acceptable if there were no negative long-term effects of estrogen therapy. But there is every indication that breast cancer rates will increase as a result of widespread long-term use of estrogen to protect women against heart disease.

> The association of estrogen use and breast cancer remains speculative, but there is evidence that long-term use ... can increase risk. ... The cancer risk posed by progestins remains speculative as well; their effect on the breast in particular is a matter of controversy and has not been the subject of adequate investigation. (OTA; *The Menopause, Hormone Therapy and Women's Health*, 40:1992)

What to do

In addition to maximizing heart health by cutting down on dietary fats, you can take Vitamin C, which has been reported to lower total cholesterol levels. Taking at least 100 IUs of vitamin E daily appears to reduce the risk of heart attack by as much as forty percent. High fiber intake is important, because fiber binds with cholesterol (in bile acids) to move it out of the system. High calcium intake improves HDL levels and, together with exercise and Vitamin D, also protects against osteoporosis. (As well, increasing milk consumption has been demonstrated to decrease blood pressure.)

Studies of men who decreased the risk of stroke by consuming aspirin have been followed up, and it has now been decided that women too can benefit. One low-dose aspirin per day, or as little as 30 mg daily, appears to reduce the threat of stroke. Coated tablets are available for those who find aspirin upsetting to the stomach.

Because these and other means of preventing heart disease – not smoking, healthy low-fat diets, exercise, and weight control – have not been evaluated, we have no idea whether nonmedical preventive strategies might be equally effective as estrogen supplementation in promoting a healthy old age. We *do* know that older women who exercise regularly and who maintain high HDL levels through the postmenopausal years have hearts and arteries typical of much younger women. More and more, we are recognizing that exercise may be the answer to a host of midlife health problems.

Breast Health

Five out of ten women see their doctors at some point in their lives about lumps, pain, swelling, or tenderness of the breasts. Pathologists have discovered that nine out of ten show some evidence of the kinds of cellular changes that we know as fibrocystic breast disease. But if nine out of ten women complain of lumpy breasts at some time or other, it must not be a *disease* at all, just part of being a woman. The fear of breast cancer can be alleviated to some degree when we recognize that lumps in the breast are normal, and that there are many different kinds of lumps. (Note, however, that susceptibility to recurring fibrocystic breast lumps, when coupled with undiagnosed digestive difficulties, may be an early warning of ovarian cancer.)

Breasts are very individual parts of the body and there are great variations in size and shape. The left breast is often larger than the right; the nipple may or may not be inverted, large or small; the surrounding area (the areola) may be pale or dark, large or small. The internal structure is similar, however, made up of milk glands, forming lobes, which converge on the nipple through a series of ducts. Fibrous bands hold the lobes apart and attach the breasts to the chest wall. The supporting fibers are responsible for the "lift," which is affected by body weight, breast size, pregnancy, and breast feeding. Age brings about a thinning out of the fibers, with fatty tissue often filling up the spaces created.

Benign breast conditions
Although we tend to think of cancer whenever we notice anything unusual about our breasts, noncancerous breast conditions are much more common. Benign breast conditions may involve changes in the

Structure of the Breast

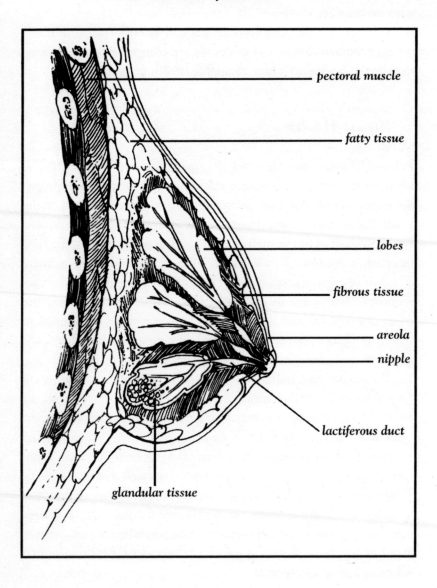

- pectoral muscle
- fatty tissue
- lobes
- fibrous tissue
- areola
- nipple
- lactiferous duct
- glandular tissue

fibrous tissue, changes in the cells of the milk ducts, or the formation of cysts. The most common is the formation of cysts (chronic mastitis). This affects approximately 30 percent of women and tends to be most bothersome between the ages thirty and forty.

At the age of thirty-eight, I discovered lumps in my breast. Convinced I had cancer, I rushed to my doctor and was given no reason to believe otherwise. My doctor suggested that the lumps were probably cancerous and made an appointment for a mammogram and biopsy. As it turned out, it was cystic mastitis. The cysts were drained and I am grateful that it wasn't worse. I've learned to do routine breast self-examination (BSE) and I feel the importance of this cannot be stressed enough. Please pass this on.

It is not known why breast cysts form, but apparently some relationship exists between fibrous tissue, diet, and stimulation by cyclical hormones. Before menopause, fluctuations in estrogen tend to produce larger, more tender cysts prior to menstruation; changes in size and sensation follow the menstrual period. Generally cysts form hard, round nodes that can be moved easily and that are filled with fluid. There may be many small ones, a few medium-sized ones, or even one large one. When they are too large and painful, they may be aspirated (drained) with a fine needle. A darkish fluid – yellow, green, or brown – is withdrawn and sent for routine analysis. Cysts are rarely cancerous: the rare cancerous cyst may have more to do with the cyst lining, which is smooth when benign and irregular when malignant. Cysts often disappear spontaneously after menopause.

Methylxamine (found in coffee, tea, cola drinks, and chocolate) seems to aggravate formation of breast cysts. Nicotine may also be a factor, since smokers seem to be more prone to cysts. Low-fat diets have helped some women to reduce the incidence and discomfort. Evening primrose oil has been used by some women with promising results. Increased levels of Vitamin A, Vitamin B_6 (50 mg daily), and Vitamin E (800 IUs daily in four doses of 200 IUs) have also been used with excellent results. (For more information about Vitamin E and some precautions about its use, see page 39.)

Changes in the fibrous tissue of the breasts can lead to a number of conditions. If a rubbery, painless tumor forms, this is a fibroadenoma. These tumors, which usually occur before age thirty-five, are not influenced by the menstrual cycle and move easily under the skin; they can usually be felt in the part of the breast closest to the armpit. A rare form of this condition may occur during menopause: giant fibroadenoma, also known as cystosarcoma phyllodes or giant myxoma. (I include all these terms just in case you have a doctor who likes to bamboozle you with big words!) In the case of giant fibroadenoma, the lump grows rapidly to a large size and must be surgically removed.

Another rare condition that may also affect menopausal women is fibrosis (not to be confused with fibrositis), or fibrous dysplasia. This consists of a firm, painless mass with no defined edges, making it difficult to feel where normal tissue stops and abnormal tissue starts. Most of these fibrous tissue abnormalities are benign.

Breast cancer is much more likely to stem from changes in the milk ducts, although even here, very few conditions are precancerous. Adenosis (which simply means abnormal growth) is a form of breast lump that may occur inside the milk duct. A lump under the nipple or areola may be caused by intraductal papillomas – wartlike growths that may produce a discharge from the nipple. An inflammation of the milk ducts, which is more common among postmenopausal women, is duct ectasia. It may also produce nipple discharge.

It is estimated that up to 10 percent of women experience nipple discharge at one time or another. Some women have a white discharge for months after a baby is weaned. Others may notice a clear, or yellow, or reddish brown discharge either occurring spontaneously or when the nipple is squeezed. Any discharge should be investigated, even though it is not unusual.

There are some serious forms of duct ectasia – plasma cell mastitis or comedomastitis. Occasionally the wartlike growths under the nipple are diagnosed as ductal papillomatosis and require intensive care. Duct hyperplasia (also known as hyperplastic disease) is a rare overgrowth of the lining of the milk ducts and is treated as a potential malignancy.

In addition to the four kinds of benign lumps already described – chronic mastitis, fibroadenoma, adenosis, and intraductal papillomas – a lump in the breast might be a lipoma (a fatty growth that can occur anywhere in the body) or fat necrosis (a hard lump resulting from a blow to the breast). Of all these kinds, textures, and sizes of breast lumps, only 10 to 15 percent will be malignant.

Breast self-examination (BSE)

Many women shy away from breast self-examination despite the promotional efforts of the Canadian Cancer Society. Unfortunately, the emphasis on BSE has been to *find lumps* rather than to become more familiar with a healthy part of the body. Most of us are very familiar with our neck and throat. We feel the neck as we adjust jewelry or fix our hair. We notice small changes – a gland swelling under the jawline, an odd bump behind the ear, a small bump, perhaps a mole, which we can feel but which is out of sight in the mirror. We monitor the state of the neck regularly and quite unself-consciously. Why can't we bring this same attitude to breast examination?

The steps involved are neither difficult nor time-consuming. Looking carefully at oneself in the mirror is easy. But the problem, for many of us, is the actual palpation – searching with the tips of the fingers for anything unusual. It is difficult to find anything unusual if one is not accustomed to the *usual*.

Many women have learned to examine their breasts while in the shower or in the tub, where soapy fingers or shower gel allow for more comfortable manipulation of breast tissue. Baby oil also helps, so you might wish to ask your doctor to use it to make breast examination more comfortable for you. When we realize that the odds are very much in our favor – that we are likely to find everything normal or a harmless condition that can be easily treated – it is easier to stick to a resolution to examine the breasts once a month.

There are no records of the incidence of benign breast conditions noticed, treated, and forgotten. But we do know that 85 to 90 percent of breast cancers are initially reported by women doing BSE, and that women who *do* examine their breasts regularly are able to notice lumps the size of the tip of a ballpoint pen, lumps much smaller than those found by experienced doctors.

Breast Self-Examination:
A New Approach

All women over 20 should practice monthly breast self-examination (BSE). Regular and complete BSE can help you find changes in your breasts that occur between clinical breast examinations (by a health professional) and mammograms.

Women should examine their breasts when they are least tender, usually seven days after the start of the menstrual period. Women who have entered menopause, are pregnant or breast feeding, and women who have silicone implants, should continue to examine their breasts once a month. Breast-feeding mothers should examine their breasts when all milk has been expressed.

If a woman discovers a lump or detects any changes, she should seek medical attention. Nine out of ten women will not develop breast cancer and most breast changes are not cancerous.

Remember the seven Ps for a complete BSE:
1. Positions 2. Perimeter 3. Palpation 4. Pressure. 5. Pattern 6. Practice and Feedback 7. Plan of Action

1. Positions

In each position look for changes in contour and texture of the breasts, color and texture of the skin and nipple, and evidence of discharge from the nipples.

arms relaxed at side

hands on hips

arms raised above head

bending forward

Palpation: Side-lying and flat. Use your left hand to palpate the right breast, while holding your arm at a right angle to the rib cage, with the elbow bent. Repeat the procedure on the other side. The side-lying position allows a woman, especially one with large breasts, to most effec-

Breast Self-Examination:

tively examine the outer half of the breast. A woman with small breasts may need only the flat position.

Side-lying position: Lie on the opposite side of the breast to be examined. Rotate the shoulder (on the same side as the breast to be examined) back to the flat surface.
Flat position: Lie flat on your back with a pillow or folded towel under the shoulder of the breast to be examined.

2. Perimeter

The examination area is bounded by a line which extends down the middle of the armpit to just beneath the breast, continues across along the underside of the breast to the middle of the breastbone, then moves up to and along the collarbone and back to the middle of the armpit. Most breast cancers occur in the upper outer area of the breast (*see shaded area in illustration*).

3. Palpation with pads of the fingers

Use the pads of three or four fingers to examine every inch of your breast tissue. Move your fingers in circles about the size of a dime. Do not lift your fingers from your breast between palpations. You can use powder or lotion to help your fingers glide from one spot to the next.

Breast Self-Examination:

4. Pressure

Use varying levels of pressure for each palpation, from light to deep, to examine the full thickness of your breast tissue. Using pressure will not injure the breast.

vertical strip

start in armpit

light medium deep

5. Pattern of search

Use one of the following search patterns to examine all of your breast tissue. Palpate carefully beneath the nipple. Any incision should also be carefully examined from end to end. Women who have had breast surgery should still examine the entire area and the incision.

Vertical strip: Start in the armpit, proceed downward to the lower boundary. Move a finger's width toward the middle and continue palpating upward until you reach the collarbone. Repeat this until you have covered all breast tissue. Make at least six strips before the nipple and four strips after the nipple. You may need between 10 and 16 strips.

Wedge: Imagine your breast divided like the spokes of a wheel. Examine each separate segment, moving from the outside boundary toward the nipple. Slide fingers back to the boundary, move over a finger's width and repeat this procedure until you have covered all breast tissue. You may need between 10 and 16 segments.

wedge

Circle: Imagine your breast as the face of a clock. Start at 12 o'clock and palpate along the boundary of each circle until you return to your starting point. Then move down a finger's width and continue palpating in ever smaller circles until you

Breast Self-Examination:

reach the nipple. Depending on the size of your breast, you may need eight to ten circles.

circle

Nipple discharge: Squeeze your nipples to check for discharge. Many women have a normal discharge.

Axillary Examination: Examine the breast tissue that extends into your armpit while your arm is relaxed at your side.

6. *Practice with Feedback*

It is important that you perform BSE while your instructor watches to be sure you are doing it correctly. Practice your skills under supervision until you feel comfortable and confident.

7. *Plan of action*

Discuss the Cancer Society breast cancer detection guidelines with your health professional.

Schedule your clinical breast examination and mammogram as appropriate.

Do monthly BSE. Ask your health professional for feedback on your BSE skills.

Report any changes to your health care professional.

Reprinted with permission from the American Cancer Society, California Division, Inc.

In January last year I had a biopsy on my right breast, which showed a carcinomic growth. To make a long story short, the cancer had spread to my spine and the blood tests showed it is a hormone-fed cancer. The clinic recommended cobalt radiation treatments to irradiate the ovaries.

Needless to say, I was fully into menopause literally overnight, with about twenty to thirty hot flushes daily. One thing I learned: if there is any visual change in your breasts – even if a lump cannot be found – get to a doctor immediately and keep going until you find a doctor who will listen to you. I had a dimple in my breast. I got worried when the doctor couldn't feel a lump. The dimple kept getting larger. Listen to your intuition, because you know your body better than anyone else, including all doctors!

Diagnosis

Because of the increased risk of breast cancer in midlife, many physicians now routinely send their patients for a mammogram. The referral to a radiology department or a clinic does *not* mean that anything unusual has been detected. If you have seen the doctor because of a lump, it may be biopsied in the doctor's office; if anything unusual shows up on the mammogram, you will be sent for a biopsy. Rather than becoming alarmed about incipient cancer, we should learn to accept mammograms and biopsies as routine procedures in the maintenance of good health. We don't panic about getting standard blood tests or chest X-rays, although each could just as easily point to some kind of abnormality. As we get older, it seems important to look at a biopsy in the same way – just one more standard test that helps to confirm our continuing good health.

There are a number of ways to examine breast tissue without breaking the skin. Thermography uses heat sensitivity to map areas where there is rapid cell growth (assumed to be tumors) and to contrast this with normal tissue. However, a mild inflammation may produce heat, so for this and other reasons, thermography has not been found to be consistently accurate. Transillumination (and a more recent offshoot of this, diaphanography) uses a bright light shining against the breast to show up darker masses of tissue. The accuracy of these methods depends on the density of the breast tissue. So far, they have been used only in conjunction with other methods although there is growing suspicion that thermography could be better utilized. Part of this is technology, part of it is political because the radiologists' associations in the U.S.A. and Canada have created a virtual monopoly on breast cancer screening.

Ultrasound, which can differentiate fluid-filled cysts from solid masses, is less reliable after menopause when the breast tissue changes (and when cysts tend to disappear anyway). Any or all of these methods may be used if a woman refuses mammography.

Menopausal women have breasts that are better suited to mammography than are the breasts of younger women. At midlife, breasts become less fibrous and more fatty, yielding the high contrasts needed for accurate diagnosis. Postmenopausal women on ET or CHT have denser breasts than women not receiving hormone therapy; increased density slightly diminishes the sensitivity of mammograms for early detection. The long-term effects of mammogram radiation may be worrisome to younger women, but by age fifty, we can afford to worry less; it is estimated that it would take at least thirty years for any radiation effects to show up. (If you are frightened of the long-term effects of radiation, you may be cheered to know that a thorough *seven- to ten-minute* clinical breast examination by a trained professional appears to be as effective as mammography – at least for women aged 50 to 59.) The potential for radiation effects is reduced as more state-of-the-art machines become available. Currently, it is recommended that a baseline mammogram be done at age fifty (some provincial cancer associations say forty), followed by regular biannual mammograms. If there is breast cancer in the immediate family, some experts recommend that examinations start at a younger age and be scheduled every year or six months.

When you schedule your mammogram, ask about the facilities: Is the equipment used solely for mammography? Is the radiation dose 0.4 rads or less? Are the technicians trained specifically in mammography? Does the radiologist who reads the plates read adequate numbers of mammograms (preferably several daily)?

The mammogram is usually conducted by a female technician in privacy and is a short procedure. Each breast is placed between two plates and pressure exerted to compress it as much as possible – once horizontally and once vertically. When a mammography is properly done, it is indeed painful but, fortunately, the pain only lasts for a few seconds. Women with larger-than-normal breasts are likely to find it uncomfortable, and the sensation of cold steel against warm flesh is not pleasant. However, the newer machines use warmer substances (plastics, for instance) and some exert the final fractions of compression automatically as the technician steps into the booth, or allow the woman herself to finish the compression. This means that the worst sensation of squeezing is very brief. If you do have the misfortune to run into an insensitive technician, be sure to complain to the person in charge.

Because postmenopausal women no longer have menstrual cycles to account for the size or tenderness of breast lumps, any lump will be treated with suspicion. In addition, because the odds of breast cancer increase with age, doctors are on the alert for any abnormality. If you report finding a lump, your doctor may want to perform a quick, wide-needle biopsy in the office. This is done using a local anesthetic (which freezes the area) and a second needle to draw out a sample of cells. Sometimes the procedure is done at an outpatient clinic.

Breast cancer

Despite the variety and frequency of benign breast conditions, to most women the term *breast health* means the avoidance of breast cancer. Because our culture views breasts primarily as symbols of femininity and sexuality (one reason that we may be reluctant to examine them), most of us harbor an irrational fear of breast cancer. We tell ourselves that we are not at risk, even though 70 to 80 percent of new cancers are diagnosed in women who are *not* in a specific risk category. This is how fear gets in the way of sensible self-care.

If your mother or a sister has (or has had) breast cancer, you are at higher-than-normal risk. If you have never been pregnant, or had your first child after age thirty, or did not breast-feed, you are at slightly higher risk than average. If you had an early menarche (first menstrual period) and a late menopause, the risk is increased. And finally, if you are overweight and eat foods high in fats, your risk is higher. Some of these risk factors cannot be changed, but they are worth knowing about – if not for you, then for the next generation.

Some years ago I had my first mammogram and it was clear. This was because my left breast inclined to be a bit fibro-cystic so nothing could be seen. A year later, there was some-thing there, but in my right breast. You couldn't feel it though. It turned out to be malignant, and during a second operation to remove a quarter of my breast, lymph-node involvement was found. I have presently had two bouts of chemotherapy, with six to go. Four years ago, my sister (who is five years younger than me) had a mammogram, which was clear. She was experiencing menopausal problems and her doctor prescribed estrogen. When they discovered that I had breast cancer, she asked for another mammogram, and sure enough, she has it too! She, like me, had a lumpectomy and is presently undergoing radiation therapy. Both our tumors were less than 1 cm (.39 in.) and the prognosis is good, but I'm afraid I feel we would never have had these cancers if it wasn't for estrogen. As soon as the cancer was diagnosed I was taken off estrogen and put on tamoxifen, an anti-estrogen. I was told the other day that my tumor has estrogen receptors. It makes me sick to think that for four years I was feeding the thing.

I should mention that my older sister has been on estro-gen for about ten years and is fine. I guess not everyone is going to get cancer from taking estrogen, but I would not wish what I have been through on anyone. I think the risk is too great.

Some breast cancers are hormone-dependent, in which case treatment is directed toward reducing hormone levels in the body as quickly and as completely as possible. Other cancers do not react to hormones, and still others appear to be a mixture of the two. There are contradictory reports about the long-term effects of oral contraceptives on breast cancer. Some say that long-term pill users are at decreased risk; some say the contrary. Synthetic estrogen in the form of diethylstilbestrol (DES) – once routinely administered to reduce the risk of miscarriage – is now known to be associated with levels of breast cancer at least 30 percent higher than normal in the women who were given it. ET is suspected to cause an increase in breast cysts and fibrous lumps, but we don't know enough about use of ET in relation to breast cancer. (For more about this, see chapter 5.)

On rare occasions, a woman may notice that her nipple is itchy, red, and weeping. It may look and feel like a simple skin infection, but home remedies such as salves and lotions won't help. It's time to see a doctor. It could be Paget's disease, a rare form of cancer (not to be confused with Paget's disease of the bone).

Because breast cancer is probably two or three different diseases (one of which may affect only postmenopausal women), there are many different treatments. If you know women who have breast cancer, you may find the differences in their treatments confusing. This does not necessarily reflect different attitudes of their doctors, but rather different types of cancer.

If you *do* find a lump in your breast and it *does* turn out to be malignant, the prospects for full recovery are better than they've ever been. About 70 percent of early-stage breast cancers are cured by surgery; the balance will require radiation and/or surgery plus drug therapy. Cancers will recur in only about one-third of the remaining 30 percent. Because most surgeons prefer to perform a lumpectomy (which removes the lump and leaves the breast virtually intact) where possible, rather than the traditional but disfiguring removal of the breast (mastectomy), the odds of losing a breast, either with or without underlying muscle and/or underarm lymph nodes, have been markedly reduced. Whether lumpectomy or mastectomy, adjuvant (drug) therapy and/or radiation treatments are also frequently recommended.

When cancer is diagnosed, try to find a strong friend to lean on. Discuss your options. If your doctor insists that you have the procedure *he* or *she* recommends, be sure to get a second opinion. (See chapter 7 for details.) Not only should you insist on a second opinion, but you should also insist on time. Women have, too often, been wheeled into an operating room not knowing whether they would emerge whole or not. It is generally conceded that even in extreme cases, women should be permitted two separate procedures – first the biopsy and later, after advice and deliberation, a second operation. Most of all, women need support and friendship to resist hasty decisions.

The incidence of *never-discovered cancer* in women over the age of seventy (who have died of other causes) is nineteen times that of discovered (palpable) breast cancer. This means that for every woman who has a breast lump diagnosed as malignant, there are nineteen women whose breast lumps never grow – lumps that appear and never get larger, or disappear, or grow so slowly that they are never noticed.

It has been belatedly recognized, for instance, that four out of five cases of *ductal carcinoma in situ* (DCIS) never develop into full-blown breast cancer. I wonder how many women have been through the whole anguishing process – surgery followed by radiation followed by chemotherapy followed by years of fearing a recurrence – because DCIS was found?

Experts believe that potentially cancerous lumps may be with us from puberty onward, when the breasts first develop, but how our immune system acts to stop these lumps from developing is still a mystery.

So breast cancer is probably not something that we "get," like a cold or the flu. Environmental factors – pollutants, chemicals, diet, even stress – undoubtedly play a part. The seeds of breast cancer are already sown in each of us and are as unpredictable and unexpected as all those other lumps – whether cysts, adenomas, adenosis, lipoma, or fat necrosis.

✦

Tamoxifen, a SERM, or anti-estrogen prescribed to reduce the risk of a recurrence, is given to women who have had an episode of breast cancer. In an effort to enlarge the market, tamoxifen has also been given to healthy women who may or may not be at risk of breast cancer. (A woman of sixty with no known risk factors is considered to be at equal risk to a woman of thirty-five with a strong family history.)

The market is growing: most women today are frightened about breast cancer because they have friends or relatives that have been touched by it. But giving healthy women a drug with many known adverse effects is not the solution. Tamoxifen loses its capacity to prevent breast cancer within a few years. At the same time, it enormously increases a woman's susceptibility to uterine cancer and dangerous blood clots.

We know that more than seven out of ten new cases of breast cancer occur in women with no known risk factors. Although deaths from breast cancer are going down, the incidence (reporting of new cases) has not decreased. Why don't we spend more time and money on research into the *causes* and *prevention* of breast cancer, rather than fixating on screening and treatment?

AstraZeneca (the major manufacturer of tamoxifen) called a big press conference not too long ago to announce an early end to a tamoxifen trial using basically healthy women. Unfortunately for them, their vaunted results were disputed by parallel research studies completed in Europe, and a careful examination of the results publicized by AstraZeneca revealed very little benefit, if any, to the women involved.

Now tamoxifen is being tested against raloxifene, another SERM (see Chapter 5), but untreated women are excluded. The results may tell you how one medication performs as compared to the other, but it will not tell you if unmedicated women are just as free from this form of cancer as women taking tamoxifen or raloxifene.

I took tamoxifen for two years after my brush with breast cancer but, aside from its other adverse effects, taking a drug that caused hot flashes now (in my mid-sixties) when I had refused a drug to alleviate hot flashes ten years ago, seemed paradoxical. I'll take my chances.

CHAPTER 7

MENOPAUSE UNDER
THE KNIFE:

COMMON SURGICAL
PROCEDURES

A lthough none of the surgical procedures described in this chapter is unique to menopause, they are procedures that the menopausal woman should know about. This is particularly true of hysterectomy, which may bring on an earlier-than-normal menopause, and oophorectomy (or ovariectomy), which causes immediate and severe menopause. If surgery is recommended, such as for heavy or irregular bleeding, women may readily agree to an operation because they're too frightened to explore other avenues. This may be one reason that such an unusually high number of operations are performed on women.

Deciding about Surgery

It is no surprise that surgery is more likely to be proposed by a surgeon than by another type of physician. Gynecologists are surgeons, and one of the strongest predictors of high rates of hysterectomy in a given area is the number of surgeons. In England, where fewer surgeons are trained as a proportion of all medical doctors, the rates for many standard surgical procedures are significantly lower. For instance, only 14 percent of English women have hysterectomies, compared with 25 to 35 percent in the United States and Canada. In fact, it is the discrepancy between rates of surgery from one country to another and from region to region within a country that has led to the widespread practice of seeking a second opinion or even third opinion before agreeing to surgery. Those of us concerned with women's health recommend that you *always* get a second opinion or third opinion if you are contemplating major surgery.

To get a second opinion, you should consult a doctor whose opinion is likely to be independent from the first. This will involve finding a doctor with a different hospital affiliation, of a different age group, with offices in a different area. Find someone who is *not* part of the same "old boys' network." A good family physician or general practitioner is more likely to consider other options before recommending "the knife." No reputable surgeon will object to a second or third opinion; if you feel you are being pressured into an operation, you should dig in your heels. The time you take to make decisions *before* surgery has a lot to do with your psychological well-being *after* surgery.

If you decide to go ahead with the surgery, you should have every confidence in the doctor who performs the operation. Sometimes it's possible to get valuable information by telephoning the operating-room nurses who assist the surgeon. Ask how many similar procedures this person has performed. You may also want to talk with some of his or her patients to find out if the doctor stays as involved and concerned *after* the operation as *before*. You have a right to this information and more. If the surgeon you have chosen is patronizing or dismisses your questions, find another doctor.

If your problem is unmanageable bleeding, whether regular (cyclical) or irregular, or an unbearable sensation of discomfort or pressure, and your doctor recommends immediate surgery (without providing an acceptable and clear rationale), you might be wise to switch to someone who will seek alternatives.

Recently I was hospitalized for severe abdominal pain with elevated temperature, pulse, and a drop in blood pressure. It was diagnosed as PID (pelvic inflammatory disease) and my gynecologist immediately recommended a hysterectomy.

Uneasy about the idea of undergoing major surgery, I con-
sulted a friend's doctor, who instead suggested that, since it
was the first flare-up, I try antibiotics. I was then treated
with high doses of intravenous antibiotics and was released
five days later. This happened four years ago this month
and I've had no recurrence. I know now it pays to get a
second opinion.

If you are postmenopausal and suddenly start to bleed, your doctor is even more likely to recommend hysterectomy, suspecting cancer. According to the latest statistics, this kind of bleeding is caused
by cancer in only 7 percent of cases – not sufficient reason to con-
sent to major surgery before other avenues are explored.

Some remedies for heavy bleeding are outlined in chapter 3.
Aside from remedies using nonprescription drugs, a number of hormonal treatments are available: danazol (Cyclomen), which is
often prescribed to women with endometriosis, and GnRH or
gonadotropin-releasing hormone analog (Lupron), both of which
are prescribed to still-menstruating women in order to induce a
pseudomenopause. This treatment may be considered beneficial
when endometriosis and/or fibroids cause heavy bleeding. Women
who are no longer ovulating but who continue to bleed irregular-
ly may be given progesterone (often Provera) to help flush out
the uterus and tide them over until the last menstrual period.
Clomiphene citrate (Clomid or Serophene, the "fertility drug") is
sometimes prescribed to reestablish ovulatory cycles. However, not
only does this drug "feed" fibroids but long-term use increases the
risks of ovarian cancer. Because there are major side effects associated with any strong drug, it is wise to inform yourself about these
before you agree to treatment. If your doctor is reluctant to discuss
side effects, check the CPS (*Compendium of Pharmaceuticals and
Specialties*) or the Canadian Medical Association's *Guide to
Prescription and Over-the-Counter Drugs* at the library or at your
pharmacy. Another handy reference is James Long's *The Essential
Guide to Prescription Drugs*.

Conditions Often Resulting in Surgery

Fibroids

The most common reason for a hysterectomy is fibroids, which are dense and harmless growths inside, outside, or between the walls of the uterus or on a stalk attached to the uterus (see p. 162). Fibroids are tolerable until they grow so large that they exert pressure on the rectum, bladder, or vagina – or until they cause pain during menstruation as the uterus attempts to expel them.

Fibroids are not usually dangerous. Because they thrive on estrogen, they become more troublesome as estrogen levels dip and soar just prior to menopause. Some women don't know they have fibroids until they start on ET, which causes the fibroids to grow. Once the last menstrual period has passed (assuming there is no hormone therapy), fibroids usually shrink and eventually disappear. For many women, the solution is to hold on for the last few years until menopause takes care of the situation. Should the fibroids become intolerable, a myomectomy (a procedure that removes the fibroids but not the uterus) may be possible.

Only very rarely does a fibroid become malignant (leiomysarcoma), but this is estimated to occur to one woman in 150,000. Do not be coerced into having a hysterectomy "because the fibroid might turn cancerous."

Several years ago, my gynecologist recommended a hysterectomy because of fibroid growth in my uterus. At the time he made no mention of alternative remedies, only that there seemed to be an increased risk of cancer if they were not removed. Terrified of even the thought of cancer, I underwent the surgery. Following the operation, I was told that he'd also removed both ovaries. When I asked why, he stated, "You're better off without them ... you have no use for them anyway!" Now that I know this condition could have been alleviated by diet, and the operation perhaps prevented had I had more information, it fills me with frustration and rage.

Fibroids may be diagnosed using a hysterogram or a sonogram. The hysterogram is frequently used if fibroids inside the uterus are suspected. A dye is put into the uterus through a tube and X-rays are taken. The sonogram is a procedure using ultrasound. Either a transducer is rubbed across the belly or, in a more sophisticated procedure, a tamponlike transducer is placed inside the vagina. In order to do a sonogram, the bladder must be full, which is often uncomfortable. However, this procedure may enable you to get a more accurate diagnosis before making an important decision about the next step.

There is speculation that fibroids may thrive on a high-fat diet. It is known that they are much more likely to occur in women who are overweight or obese and that the risk increases with each substantial weight gain. Anecdotal information, although scientifically suspect, tells us that some women have reduced and eliminated fibroids by switching to a diet very low in fats – for example, a macrobiotic diet or the Pritikin Diet. (A low-fat intake may also help alleviate fibrocystic breast disease.)

Endometriosis

This condition accounts for about one-fifth of all hysterectomies. For some unknown reason (exposure to dioxins is suspected), cells of the lining of the uterus (the endometrium) migrate outside the uterus and lodge inside the pelvic cavity – on the ovaries, fallopian tubes, bladder, or rectum. Slight endometriosis may go undetected because the cells are all but invisible in the early stages. However, larger clumps of cells tend to respond to the estrogen/progesterone of the normal menstrual cycle, swelling, bleeding, and causing intense pain because the blood cannot escape in the usual way. These clumps of cells eventually blacken and take on the appearance of burn sites inside the abdomen. Endometriosis is commonly found in women between the ages of thirty and forty, although it has been diagnosed in women of all ages. A woman often consults a number of doctors before the condition is correctly diagnosed.

Because endometriosis disappears during pregnancy, drugs that induce a false pregnancy or false menopause may provide some relief. Depending on age, a woman may be given oral contraceptives; danazol (Cyclomen), a drug that mimics a weak androgen (hormone produced by the adrenal glands); or leuprolide, a GnRH or gonadotropin-releasing hormone analog (Lupron). There are potential side effects to any drug (e.g., danazol has negative effects on blood fats and GnRH analogs may affect bone strength), but it is worth investigating drug therapy before resorting to surgery. At the same time, the doctor may use a laparoscopy (a fiber-optic technique) to investigate the extent of the damage.

Like a D&C, a laparoscopy may be either diagnostic or operative. If the diagnosis is confirmed, cauterization or lasers may be used to burn away sites of errant cells or to remove the entire peritoneum (lining of the pelvic cavity). Laparotomy, a related but more extensive procedure, may also be indicated. Neither of these procedures will cure endometriosis, but they "buy time," both for the woman who wishes to conceive and for the woman approaching natural menopause. Laparoscopy requires an overnight stay in hospital and may be repeated with no untoward effects.

> I am thirty-six years old. Three weeks ago, I underwent
> surgery to remove a 10 cm (4 in.) cyst on my left ovary.
> This ovary was finally also removed, as they discovered I
> had a severe case of endometriosis. Several cysts were also
> burned off the right ovary and my doctor says I now have a
> 50 percent chance of recurrence, at which time my uterus,
> remaining ovary, and tubes will probably have to be removed
> – causing instant menopause.

According to the Endometriosis Association, hysterectomy is an effective remedy in only a minority of cases. Eighty-five percent of women continue to have problems after the operation, even when ET is withheld. (Many doctors suggest that ET be introduced after an interval of a few months. This means that when ovarian function is affected – as happens in one-third to one-half of cases – the patient may experience the effects of menopause immediately after the operation.) If all else has failed, a hysterectomy and bilateral salpingo-oophorectomy (removal of the uterus, ovaries, and fallopian tubes) may be suggested. Even after this procedure, 5 percent of endometriosis sufferers will experience a recurrence.

Adenomyosis

This condition is similar to endometriosis and also accounts for about one-fifth of all hysterectomies. In a case of adenomyosis, endometrial cells move into the muscles of the uterus, causing the uterus to enlarge and harden. Menstruation then becomes very heavy and very painful. However, adenomyosis remains undetected in about 30 percent of cases and is discovered only when surgery is performed for another reason. Adenomyosis usually occurs in women who have had more than one pregnancy and who are between the ages of forty and fifty. It is rare after menopause.

> Two years ago, I began experiencing extremely heavy bleeding during my periods. They had always been fairly light and painless, but gradually I became so incapacitated by the pain, I couldn't go to work for two days each month. I was also using about three or four more tampons every day. I consulted my doctor, who suggested a D&C. He suspected I had a condition called adenomyosis, so I had a hysterectomy a month later. It turned out he was right. Although my recovery has been slow and difficult, I am now better able to function and no longer have to dread that "time of the month."

Prolapse

Most of us think of uterus when we hear the word *prolapse*, although uterine prolapse is only one form. The word simply means the downward displacement of an organ or part. Prolapse may affect the uterus, the bladder, the urethra, or the rectum.

According to one well-known English doctor, about one woman in five attending her clinic has some form of uterine prolapse. This means that the uterus begins to descend into the vagina (this is *not* the same as a "tipped" uterus, which does not need correction). In extreme cases of prolapse, the uterus may protrude from the mouth of the vagina. Weakened pelvic muscles, as a result of many pregnancies or obesity, are often responsible.

Different Types of Prolapse

bladder

spine

colon

uterus

cervix

rectum

vagina

urethra

prolapse of uterus

vaginal pessary

prolapse of bladder (cystocele)
prolapse of urethra (urethocele)

prolapse of rectum (rectocele)

urethocele   cystocele

rectocele

The discomfort of an extreme uterine prolapse may be relieved by the insertion of a pessary, a device that lifts the uterus out of the vagina. While the pessary is in place, a strict and regular routine of

Kegel exercises should be adopted (see page 45) and, if necessary, a weight-loss program as well. Some women have found that yoga exercises are helpful, especially the shoulder stand. If this doesn't work, a minor operation called a suspension may be performed, provided the muscles are in shape. If the uterus is normal (this can be checked using a hysteroscope), surgical suspension is infinitely preferable to hysterectomy.

If hysterectomy is warranted, it will usually be done through the vagina, using the lithotomy position (similar to that used during a Pap smear). The ovaries and fallopian tubes are left intact, which eliminates the necessity of an incision. However, the operating table is often rotated into a near-vertical position so that the surgeon can more easily see what he or she is doing. Because the table is tilted only after the patient is anesthetized, many women wonder why they experience severe backache after the operation. This operation is also more likely to incur damage to the bladder, ureters, or the nerves affecting bowel and bladder function, compared with an abdominal hysterectomy. Such damage may cause the involuntary passing of small amounts of urine. This can be relieved by faithful repetitions of Kegel exercises or through a minor surgical procedure, a colporrhapy, which tightens the support around the urethra (the tube that carries urine out of the body) and takes pressure off the vaginal wall.

Prolapse, whether of the uterus, bladder, urethra or rectum, can also be relieved by exercise and diet, before a final decision about surgery is required. Doctors have noticed that the incidence of prolapse is decreasing, perhaps because women are having fewer children or perhaps because their muscles are stronger, since they are exercising more.

Cervical abnormalities

The cervix, or bottom third of the uterus, is prone to a number of conditions that, if not watched closely or left untreated, can develop into something serious. Cervicitis is usually detected by means of an unusual discharge – unusual in color, texture, or aroma – a signal to make an appointment with a doctor. Or you may be told of some abnormality as the result of a routine Pap test.

Depending on the results of your Pap test, you may be referred for colposcopy. A colposcope is a special microscope that permits magnification of the cervix by ten to forty times. If suspicious cells are found, samples are scraped for biopsy. The examination takes fifteen to twenty minutes and is uncomfortable but not painful. If the biopsy is not conclusive, more tissue will be needed. Cells of the cervix may be removed using a "punch" (like the kind used to make a perforation in paper). There are no nerves in the cervix, so this is uncomfortable but not terribly painful, although severe uterine cramps may follow. (Don't plan to go back to work the same day!)

A more comprehensive sample of cells requires a cone biopsy, which entails a general anesthetic and hospital admission in order to remove a cone-shaped section of the cervix. This is done so that cells deeper inside the cervix can be examined. Sometimes the cone is enough to arrest any abnormality. Although some cancers of the cervix have been halted using this procedure, conization is relatively rare these days. There is a tendency for the cervix to close up as a result of the procedure, so the consequences of conization are more critical for women who wish to become pregnant. This may not be an issue for women approaching menopause. Results of the biopsy (punch or cone) vary according to the depth and extent of abnormal cells. If the abnormality is minor, a stiff brush may be enough to remove the offending cells and induce the cervix to regrow normally. If not, cryosurgery or laser surgery may be recommended.

Loop electrosurgical excision procedure (or LEEP) is a procedure that eliminates the two steps of biopsy and then surgery. LEEP uses a low-voltage electrified wire loop to cut out the abnormal tissue and at the same time preserve it for biopsy. It is helpful in confirming the type and extent of the abnormality, and can be performed in a matter of minutes in a doctor's office. The only concern is that the ease of the procedure may lead to abuse. Make sure that you have had a colposcopy first and that overgrowth of cells on the cervix (or CIN – *cervical intraepithelial neoplasia*) has been established.

In cryosurgery, no anesthetic is needed. The cells on the surface of the cervix are frozen using a probe that directs a solution onto them; these surface cells turn white and soon start to slough off. This procedure is uncomfortable but not painful. The process is certainly preferable to more drastic forms of surgery, although it results in a watery discharge for days or weeks afterward and the discharge can become foul smelling at times. But eventually the surface of the cervix grows new and normal cells.

Laser surgery, which has become increasingly popular during the past few years, vaporizes abnormal cervical tissue; it is preferred by many gynecologists who have invested in expensive laser equipment.

Each of these three procedures – LEEP, cryosurgery, and laser – is equally effective, and the choice may simply come with the surgeon. It is worthwhile to inquire about the advantages and disadvantages of each, for your particular case, before consenting. This may involve talking to three different doctors.

Known risk factors for CIN are young age at first intercourse, multiple male sex partners, failure to have regular Pap tests, and smoking. (The nicotine found in the vaginal secretions of cigarette smokers is in concentrations forty times higher than in the blood.)

Some cervical conditions prompt remedial action, but hysterectomy is rarely warranted. Even when a diagnosis of early carcinoma in situ (malignant cells confined to the surface) is made, steps can be taken to head off further trouble, without resorting to hysterectomy. Choose your doctor carefully. Find someone with a conservative approach, someone who views major surgery as a last resort.

Pelvic inflammatory disease (PID)

PID is a general term used to cover a variety of inflammations that may affect the pelvic cavity. Use of an intrauterine device (IUD) for birth control, coupled with an increase in sexual activity (often with many partners), appears to have contributed to a higher incidence of PID. PID is often confused with sexually transmitted diseases (STD) – once known as venereal disease (VD) – but the causes of PID are more mysterious. It can happen to anyone. The symptoms may be pelvic pain with or without unusual bleeding, but unlike other conditions, there is often high fever during the acute phase. Most cases of PID respond to diligent treatment with antibiotics, but one episode of PID should be a signal for a woman to find and hold on to a good gynecologist.

PID can lead to a greater possibility of infertility or fertility problems, usually as a result of scarring of the fallopian tubes. Drastic surgery may be required if PID continues.

Endometrial abnormalities

Some women are frightened into having a hysterectomy as a result of a routine Pap test that indicates unusual cells within the uterus. When this happens, the cells may be identified as: (1) hyperplasia or hyperplastic; (2) cystic hyperplasia; (3) atypical adenomatous hyperplasia; or (4) carcinoma in situ.

Hyperplasia means an abnormal number of cells. It can occur naturally, or as a result of prolonged and/or heavy use of estrogen without added progesterone, or as a result of using tamoxifen. Each of these hyperplasias is a step toward uterine cancer, but none is serious enough to warrant an immediate hysterectomy. Even carcinoma in situ, frightening as it may sound, means cancerous cells that are restricted to one location; thus it may be possible to remove the cells without removing the uterus. Endometrial cancer has a high cure rate because most forms are extremely slow growing. (The exception may be endometrial cancer due to tamoxifen use; this is under investigation.) Any condition described to you as "precancerous" (or in similar words) is unnecessarily alarming. After all, there's not one cell in the entire body that isn't "precancerous."

A number of steps can be taken to change the characteristics of the endometrial cells – among them a course of progesterone and one or more D&Cs. Don't assume that you are simply postponing the inevitable and agree to an unnecessary operation. Always look at the alternatives to major surgery.

After two years without a menstrual period, I developed some vaginal bleeding. I had been on estrogen for about six years, so my gynecologist immediately stopped the hormones and told me to come back if there was any more "breakthrough bleeding" (as he called it) and he would do a D&C. I tried to ignore the slight bleeding for several months and then finally booked for a D&C. The results showed endometrial hyperplasia with atypical cells. According to the doctor, I now had several choices. One was to wait for more bleeding, then another D&C and, if cells had worsened, to have a hysterectomy. The second choice was to have a hysterectomy immediately. He recommended the second option.

After consulting several other doctors (including a young, recently graduated female gynecologist) who all recommended the second option, I decided to go ahead with the surgery. I feel one hundred percent better than before surgery and would like to start losing weight, exercising, and being generally more careful about my health. I would also like to stop taking estrogen, which I began again after surgery, but for now it is very necessary.

I went for a six-week checkup last week and everything has healed perfectly. When I asked if I should come back for a further check, the doctor said, "There's no need to come and see me. You have nothing for me to examine."

Surgical Procedures

Dilatation and curettage (D&C)

This minor operation is often ordered to control extensive bleeding (menorrhagia) when drug therapy has been unsuccessful. Dilatation opens up the uterus for inspection. The curette is a long, spoon-handled instrument that is used to scrape out the tissues lining the uterus.

A D&C may be warranted to better diagnose a problem – for instance, following an abnormal Pap test – or when adenomyosis (endometrial cells enlarging the uterus) is suspected. Sometimes a minor procedure such as this, or even a Pap test or punch biopsy, may prod the uterus into regulating itself. Aside from its diagnostic value, a D&C can also relieve uterine polyps (harmless, pod-shaped growths) or submucous fibroids. If the polyps or fibroids recur, a second or third D&C may eliminate the need for major surgery.

Dilatation and Curettage

Because the D&C is a minor procedure, it is sometimes done in an outpatient clinic. The patient reports early in the morning and is discharged that evening. When the procedure is performed under general anesthetic, an overnight stay may be required. Scarring of the uterus may result, and for this reason, the D&C or a series of D&Cs may not be the best option for women wanting a child. For most menopausal women, however, these consequences are not so important.

Hysteroscopy and laser ablation

An alternative to a D&C is laser ablation of the endometrium, which may be effective when hormone treatment and/or D&Cs have been ineffective in halting severe bleeding. This procedure allows the surgeon to view the inside of the uterus using a fiber-optic device called a hysteroscope, and to destroy the deepest layer of the endometrium (lining of the uterus) either by vaporizing it with a laser or by cutting it away with a razor or a roller ball (a resectoscope). In either case, the endometrium will not grow back.

This procedure involves a short recovery period (like that for a D&C) and has no negative effects on sexual response (compared with hysterectomy). Its success rate is encouraging. The advantage of the hysteroscope is that the surgeon can see into the uterus, whereas a D&C is essentially a blind operation. It is estimated that hysteroscopy eliminates the need for unnecessary surgery in 60 to 85 percent of cases. If hysteroscopy is combined with another procedure, such as endometrial ablation, however, this will induce sterility (unlike a D&C).

Hysteroscopy and laser ablation may not be appropriate for some atypical cell changes inside the uterus (hyperplasia, etc.) or for pelvic inflammatory disease (PID). Not all surgeons have adapted to the hysteroscope and use it regularly in their practice. Still, there is good reason to shop around for someone who *is* experienced and to insist on it if it is appropriate to your situation.

Myomectomy

Myomectomy (or leiomyomectomy) is a procedure that is relatively rare in this country as opposed to England and Western Europe, although informed health consumers are helping to make it more available. A myomectomy is an operation that removes fibroids (benign tumors known as myomas or leiomyomas) but that leaves the uterus intact. The reason it is *not* more common in North America is that doctors have been trained to think of the uterus as an unnecessary organ (except for childbearing), and most are not trained or experienced in the myomectomy procedure, which often involves more bleeding and requires more patience, time, and attention to detail than does a hysterectomy.

Fibroids of different shapes and sizes are fairly common. About 20 to 30 percent of women harbor detectable fibroids, although only about a third will be bothered by them – experience abnormal bleeding, irregular menstrual periods, or feelings of pressure. Pathologists report that more than 50 percent of women have never-detected fibroids of some kind, some so tiny as to be almost invisible during autopsy.

Surgeons who perform myomectomies remove an average of 16 to 20 per operation. The fibroids recur in a small minority (10 to 20 percent) of cases. However, fibroids feed on estrogen and tend to

Fibroids In and Around the Uterus

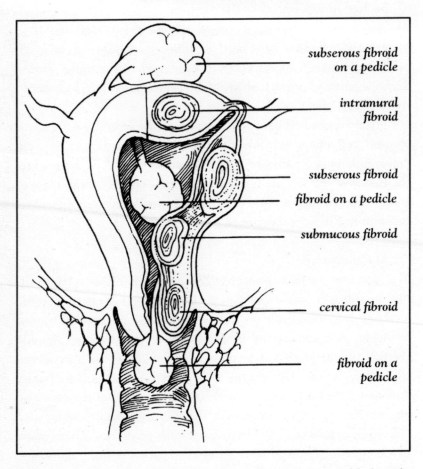

subserous fibroid
on a pedicle

intramural
fibroid

subserous fibroid

fibroid on a pedicle

submucous fibroid

cervical fibroid

fibroid on a
pedicle

shrink as one approaches menopause. If you are troubled with fibroids and wish to avoid having a hysterectomy, it may be advisable to seek out a surgeon who will agree to perform a myomectomy. Because most surgeons prefer to reserve this procedure for women who wish to retain the possibility of pregnancy, your request will be taken more seriously if you are of childbearing age.

I just received a letter from my sister in England; I had written to her about my upcoming surgery. Four months ago, my gynecologist informed me that I have uterine fibroids and I am due to have a hysterectomy two weeks from tomorrow. Yet my sister seems to feel that a hysterectomy might be unnecessary. She sent me a newspaper clipping, which states that there is an operation called "myomectomy" that involves removing only the fibroids and not the uterus. I've since spoken to two doctors. Neither had any information about or support for this procedure. I am outraged at their attitudes! They seem to feel that my uterus is of very little importance. I happen to care about it.

Hysterectomy

The word means "removal of the uterus," although it is often (and mistakenly) used to refer to removal of the ovaries as well as the uterus. When doctors speak about a hysterectomy or a TAH (total abdominal hysterectomy), they mean removal of the uterus and cervix. A partial hysterectomy (rare in North America) removes the uterus and leaves a cervical stump. A radical hysterectomy or modified radical hysterectomy involves lymph nodes outside the uterus and often entails a longer recovery with potentially more complications.

Hysterectomies are performed for a number of reasons, not all valid. When three women are hysterectomized in one area of the country for every two in another, it may be inferred that hysterectomies are still being used as the "easy" solution to a problem, rather than as an operation of last resort. Some women continue to assume that once childbearing is finished, a hysterectomy is part of the routine. Misinformation or lack of information contributes to an inflated rate of hysterectomy.

Some surgeons routinely recommend a hysterectomy for heavy bleeding without attempting preliminary measures, or neglect to tell women that fibroids tend to diminish and disappear with menopause. There is often a significant difference between a male surgeon's view of your uterus and your feelings about it. A striking example of this can be found in the hysterectomy rates in Switzerland, where female gynecologists perform half as many hysterectomies as do their male counterparts. If you feel attached to your uterus (as many of us do!), make this clear to your doctor. If the doctor is appropriate for your needs, he or she will be willing to discuss options other than surgery.

◆

Different Types of Hysterectomy

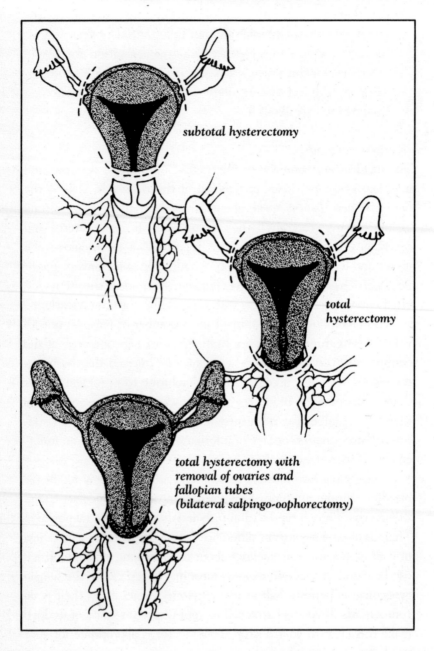

subtotal hysterectomy

total
hysterectomy

total hysterectomy with
removal of ovaries and
fallopian tubes
(bilateral salpingo-oophorectomy)

Despite the fact that medical texts and journals continue to document the adverse effects of hysterectomies, few women are told about the possibility of earlier menopause as a result of the surgery. Even when ovaries are being removed, surgeons are reluctant to mention the effects this might have on sex drive or on sexual response. Most patients believe that taking hormones will be an easy and fail-safe way to compensate for any losses resulting from the surgery. Far too many women are ill-prepared for the aftermath of the operation.

Postoperative complications affect from 10 to 25 percent of patients, particularly those who experience a radical hysterectomy. A significant number of those affected require rehospitalization. Urinary-tract infections become much more common, and for premenopausal women, the prospect of premature menopause becomes a distinct possibility, a fact that very few women are aware of. Because the ovaries are moved inside the pelvic cavity, disrupting the blood flow carrying essential hormones, ovarian function is often affected. High levels of estrogen circulating in the bloodstream during the menstruating years help to protect against heart disease and osteoporosis. When ovaries falter as a result of hysterectomy, the risks of heart disease and osteoporosis increase.

Depression follows hysterectomy in from 30 to 50 percent of cases – some studies say 70 percent. Usually this is a minor and short-term depression (such as after childbirth), but it is now being recognized that there is a biochemical source for this depression. It is not due to the trauma of anesthesia or surgery, because the effects are quite different from the experiences of women who have had appendectomies or cholecystectomies (gallbladder surgery).

Hysterectomy may permanently diminish the experience of orgasm, not only because it removes the source of prostacyclin, which is a potent vasodilator produced in the uterus, but because it amputates the cervix, rich in nerve cells that react to penile thrusting, and eliminates the pleasurable throbbing of the uterus, which often accompanies orgasm: Scar tissue at the end of the vagina may inhibit the ballooning characteristic of the vaginal barrel during orgasm; the woman may have to use a dilator to stretch the vagina and to plan, with her partner, sexual activity that will gradually make intercourse more pleasurable. (If the ovaries are also removed during a hysterectomy, both sexual desire and the capacity for response may disappear.)

Estrogen can never recreate the hormonal milieu, although it works better for some women than others. (Women are told that drugs will "replace" lost estrogen but not about the high levels of gonadotropins – FSH and LH – that appear after surgery and that may have unpredictable consequences. Nor are they told about increased risks of osteoporosis and heart disease that result.) It is impossible to predict how effective supplementary hormones will be for a particular patient. Most women find that it takes a full year to feel totally well, but some spend years trying different forms of replacement therapy in an unsuccessful effort to recapture the sensation of being well. Women are not likely to hear much about this from their surgeon.

If you decide to proceed with a hysterectomy, minimize the surprises by learning as much as you can about the operation. Recovery is often longer and more difficult if the operation is scheduled during the two weeks prior to menstruation, so plan accordingly. If your doctor is not particularly forthcoming, this may be the time to think about switching. Too many women are persuaded to stick with "experienced technicians" who are incapable of communicating effectively with their patients. Is that what you really want? Inquire about the tests required in advance, the types of anesthetic used, the location of the incision, the presurgery routine (enema? shave?), and the postsurgery possibilities (catheter? IV [intravenous]? drains? lung expansion exercises?). Examine the release forms you will be asked to sign and discuss contingencies with your doctor. When might you be expected to get up? to walk? to go home?

There are a great many women who find the quality of life much improved after a hysterectomy and who are very glad the decision was made. Research has shown that the outcome of a hysterectomy is favorable when the patient has had a few months to consider the possibilities and when she has a very clear idea of the reasons for, and techniques used, in the chosen procedure, the postsurgery routine, and the detailed steps toward full recuperation. No self-respecting surgeon objects to a second opinion, or even a third, and each consultant is likely to contribute to a more accurate picture.

A woman who views hysterectomy as a solution to extreme discomfort or continual pain will not be dissuaded by this list of "things to think about," and rightly so. For every positive experience, however, there are many women confused and miserable after their operations. The rate of hysterectomy is much higher among poorly educated women with blue-collar or low-status jobs, *because* these women have neither the opportunity nor the encouragement to consider other possibilities. This is why those interested in women's health urge caution and deliberation.

Oophorectomy (or ovariectomy)

These are the correct terms for removal of an ovary. When both ovaries are removed, it is called a bilateral oophorectomy. When the fallopian tubes are also removed (as is often the case), it's called a bilateral salpingectomy – which doctors often refer to as a BSO (*bilateral salpingo-oophorectomy*). Women who have had this operation are referred to by physicians as "castrates."

Removal of all ovarian tissue causes an immediate menopause in any menstruating woman. Removal of most ovarian tissue is often followed by menopause either because of the trauma (shock) of the surgery or because of a disturbance in the blood supply around the ovaries, which carries the hormones produced by ovarian tissue. This interruption to the cycle often brings on premature menopause. Theoretically one small part of the ovary can produce hormones sufficient to keep the cycle regular until natural menopause. In practice, however, the outcome is unpredictable.

Many gynecology textbooks still advocate the removal of healthy ovaries from any woman over forty. The shocking news is that this recommendation is based on a false statistic that has been published in textbook after textbook.* It's not surprising that surgeons who graduated ten, twenty, or thirty years ago may still adhere to this recommendation; others routinely remove ovaries when performing a hysterectomy on a woman over forty-five. This is done to avoid the possibility of ovarian cancer, a particularly lethal form of cancer that is difficult to detect and that, unlike uterine or endometrial cancer, takes hold very quickly. It is now recognized, however, that removal of the ovaries prior to natural menopause significantly increases the risks of both heart disease and osteoporosis. And the risks of heart disease and osteoporosis are incurred for *every* woman who loses ovarian tissue in order to protect the *rare* woman who will develop ovarian cancer. It is ironic that the practice of removing the ovaries in any woman over forty has led to inflated rates of heart disease and osteoporosis among older women, who are then prescribed estrogen, a medical treatment, to alleviate a condition induced by a medical procedure.

The risk of ovarian cancer in the population at large is roughly one in every one hundred (with the exception of families that have a strong history of this disease). This risk also holds for women who have had hysterectomies. Moreover, there is a suggestion that the risk may be reduced for these women, since ovaries that are found to be healthy during surgery are likely to remain healthy. Removing one healthy ovary, or all but part of one ovary, is a highly questionable practice, because as long as *any* ovarian tissue is present, the potential for ovarian cancer remains the same.

There is considerable evidence that aging ovaries still produce testosterone (vital in maintaining sex drive and a feeling of well-

---

* A medical text published in 1955 stated that, among women who had developed ovarian cancer, 4 to 4.5 percent had previously had a hysterectomy. In later years and later textbooks, this statistic was transposed to read that hysterectomized women stood a 4 to 4.5 percent chance of *developing* ovarian cancer. This error led to the mistaken belief that hysterectomy increased the risks of ovarian cancer, and has no doubt been the rationale for the removal of countless ovaries. In fact, the risk of ovarian cancer is not affected by the presence or absence of the uterus. (Cutler, 1988:105)

being) and a substance that is converted to estrone, which, in turn, helps to maintain bone strength. Choose a surgeon who is cognizant of a woman's enduring need for her ovaries. If the presence of an ovarian cyst requires investigative surgery, the patient and her surgeon should have a clear understanding that oophorectomy should not take place unless malignancy is found. This requires complete trust in your surgeon.

Prostate cancer in men is about as common and about as lethal as cancer of the ovaries in women. However, prostatectomies (the equivalent procedure for the male, which often results in impotence) are not routinely performed in order to protect them from prostate cancer. Women's health activists continue to protest the practice of removing healthy ovaries.

◆

Hysterectomy (and oophorectomy, where warranted) may now be performed using laparoscopic surgery. This is a procedure that is performed abdominally and/or vaginally, using small incisions in the abdomen – one through which the surgeon views the operating area and one or more in which instruments are inserted. The material to be removed (fibroids, uterus, fallopian tubes, ovaries) must be cut into pieces small enough to pull out through the incisions or through the vagina.

Few surgeons are experienced with laparoscopic techniques, and not every woman will be a suitable candidate. Where appropriate, however, laparoscopic hysterectomies promise a shorter recovery period and the possibility of fewer post-operative complications.

As this new procedure becomes better known, women may be more easily persuaded to choose surgery rather than alternative, non-surgical solutions for their gynecological problems. I hope that the growing availability of laparoscopic hysterectomy will not add to the current inflated incidence of hysterectomies and oophorectomies.

Cholecystectomy (removal of the gallbladder)
Gallstones are hardened bits of cholesterol, calcium, and/or bile pigments, often detected only during other surgery (often hysterectomy) or when ultrasound or CAT scans are used for some other purpose. (A

The Occurrence of Gallstones

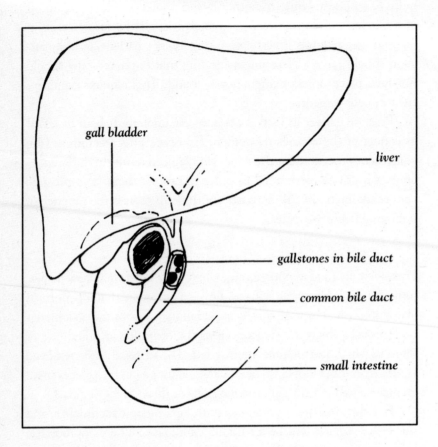

gall bladder

liver

gallstones in bile duct

common bile duct

small intestine

CAT scan may, for instance, have been ordered for suspected osteo-porosis.) Cholecystectomy, an operation to remove gallstones, is per-formed three times more often on women than on men.

The gallbladder is a storage facility for bile, the enzyme that is manufactured in the liver and directed toward the small intestine to help in the breakdown of ingested fats. A gallstone may tumble into the biliary duct, which transports this bile, lodge there (producing great pain), or cause an infection.

If you are overweight, over forty, and have had several chil-dren, you're in a high-risk category. Certain ethnic groups are also more prone to gallstone problems (e.g., Spaniards, Swedes, First Nations people), although no one has figured out if this is heredity or diet. Additional risk factors are diabetes, cirrhosis of the liver (from high alcohol consumption), and use of certain types of diuretics (thiazide derivatives). Women vulnerable to gallbladder attacks are advised to stick to a low-fat diet to minimize the possibility of such an occurrence.

Pathologists tell us that one woman in five has gallstones when she dies, although they may never have given her problems. These stones may be "silent," or asymptomatic (without symptoms). Doctors treat these differently from quiescent gallstones, which *do* cause symptoms that are likely to recur.

Because the risk of gallstones increases with use of oral contraceptives (particularly among very young women), oral estrogen is usually not recommended for women susceptible to gallstones. Obese women fall into this category because they already produce higher-than-normal amounts of estrone, a form of estrogen.

I am writing to you because I want to share my experience with other women. Last month, I was told I had gallstones and surgery was advised. After having asked around a little, I discovered that the estrogen I've been taking to deal with menopause symptoms may very well have stimulated growth of the stones. I have stopped the estrogen and have gone on a low fat diet. So far, all is well.

There are a number of nonsurgical interventions for gallstones; these include pills that dissolve stones, drips that introduce a solvent directly into the gallbladder, shock waves intended to pulverize the stones (lithotripsy), and a laparoscopic procedure. The pills have worked well on cholesterol stones, but less well on other kinds of stones (and it is impossible to analyze the stones until they are *removed*). The drip must reach the precise site of the stones (a highly specialized maneuver) because it is toxic and could damage other organs. The shock waves, which are used more successfully on kidney stones, may harm nearby lung tissue and must be administered under general anesthetic. And although laparoscopy has become popular (and easy to sell) because of the small incisions and quicker recovery period, complications are far more likely than with the traditional "open" surgical field. It pays to get precise figures on the risks accompanying each procedure.

There has been some speculation that increased rates of surgery may result from unnecessary medical intervention in asymptomatic gallstones. Reports suggest that both asymptomatic and quiescent stones require observation only, and that complications arise in just a small minority of patients. In one study where candidates with quiescent stones were followed very closely, the pain actually decreased after five years. Most doctors had assumed that it would get worse.

Some gallbladder operations are recommended because of continuing flatulence (gas) and dyspepsia (heartburn/indigestion), presumed to be caused by gallstones. Studies have shown very little relationship between these symptoms and the presence of gallstones. Even after the operations have been performed, the symptoms tend to reappear.

The best insurance against gallbladder surgery appears to be a low-fat, high-fiber diet and guarding against excessive weight gain. (Gallbladder problems have also occurred as a result of very sudden and severe weight loss.) Since gallbladder problems appear to be related to a higher risk of heart attack, the low-fat diet advocated in chapter 8 may help to reduce the risk of a number of diseases of midlife, including fibroids, gallstones, and breast cancer.

◆

The prospect of surgery is rarely pleasant and few people are wheeled in smiling to the operating room. It helps to have the support and counsel of someone we trust when making decisions about elective surgery. It helps too if the support comes from someone who understands how a woman feels about her body. Women's health organizations are doing a superb job in locating and circulating information about surgical procedures. Some are also attempting to provide an advocate for the frightened woman contemplating surgery; this advocate is a woman who will sit in on discussions with the doctor, ask pertinent questions, bolster the morale of the woman faced with a decision, and safeguard her rights. It is a role that each of us can play for one another.

PREPARING FOR MENOPAUSE:

NUTRITION AND EXERCISE

There are a number of ways to experience an uneventful menopause. One is to be born into a society where menopausal ailments are virtually unknown – in a country such as Japan, for instance, where a term for hot flashes is nonexistent. We don't know whether this stress-free menopause is due to culture, to race, or to diet. Another way is to adhere to a well-balanced vegetarian diet, to avoid alcohol, caffeine, and cigarettes, and to be in the habit of exerting oneself physically. There is speculation that multiple pregnancies and long periods of breast feeding protect against severe menopausal ailments. Perhaps the female body is not evolving speedily enough to adjust to the frequent menstrual cycles typical of a society that has recently learned how to use efficient contraception.

We cannot change our evolutionary or personal history. If we want to minimize menopausal distress, we should pay attention to nutrition and fitness before menopause arrives. We may also want to reconsider our attitudes toward menopause (and toward aging). The sting of menopause may not derive so much from physiological effects as from the negative connotations that we permit. Now is the time to rid menopause of its mystique, to view it as just one more rung on the ladder of life. The view from the top of the ladder is great, but you have to be fit enough to get there.

Your premenopausal years may be punctuated by a few bizarre and annoying changes that perhaps send you to the doctor. One that bothered me, for instance, was a change in bowel movements – a change so startling that I made an appointment with the doctor and readily agreed to a barium enema. At age forty-five, menopause never entered my mind. Because there had been no radical changes in what I regularly ate, it never occurred to me to experiment a little to see if my body had changed its way of processing certain foods. I knew nothing about menopause, and I suspect my doctor knew very little about nutrition.

> Prior to the onset of menopause, I found I was having problems with my digestion. I enjoyed red meat (loved roast beef!), lots of carbohydrates, and spicy foods. All of a sudden, I realized that my all-time favorites were giving me heartburn, indigestion, diarrhea, etc. It wasn't until my periods stopped that I made the connection. I've gradually altered my diet to include more vegetables, fruits, chicken, and now have very few digestion problems.
>
> Menopause reminds me of another similar change in my life – puberty! At thirteen or fourteen, I began to acquire a taste for foods that I had previously disliked. Now, at fifty-one, my tastes are changing again. And there's as much to look forward to with *this* change of life as there was with the last one!

The basics of good nutrition are usually self-taught. Unless we have advanced training or have had a lifelong interest in diet, we probably don't know very much. We can't look to physicians for information, because medical training tends to concentrate on pathological dietary deficiencies such as scurvy or rickets. It is not surprising that so few doctors consider diet when seeking solutions to a medical problem. Dietitians, on the other hand, view proper nutrition as the sane approach to the prevention of a host of modern-day malaises, and recent cross-cultural data (gleaned by epidemiologists) have added weight to this perspective. Diet appears to be the major factor in the low incidence of breast cancer among Japanese women and the virtual absence of cardiovascular disease among the Inuit.

Not only must we be reeducated in terms of nutrition, but we must also take a whole new look at the benefits of exercise. For too long, physical activity has been considered a distasteful way to lose inches or perhaps pounds. During the past twenty years, however, we have witnessed a revolution – exercise as the route to fitness rather than solely as a way of slimming. Women who have incorporated exercise into their lives discover that they can't do without it. More and more, exercise is proving to be the panacea we have been looking for – a way to reduce the intensity of hot flashes, to ward off the effects of depression, to find time to be by oneself, to keep one's weight at a sensible level, to ensure restorative sleep, to prevent the ravages of osteoporosis, and to minimize the risks of cardiovascular disease. The relationship between diet/exercise and maintenance of good health becomes more and more evident. If menopause is on *your* horizon and you want to manage it well, there is a great deal you can do to prepare for it.

Nutrition in Midlife

I have weighed between 130 and 135 pounds since I was about twenty-five years old. I am now forty-nine. Two years ago, my weight soared – within a period of five months – to 170. Needless to say, I was devastated and set out to find an appropriate diet. Until six months ago, absolutely nothing helped. I tried almost every diet I could get my hands on. I spoke to two doctors, both of whom said, "Menopause," but neither offered any help. They seemed to feel it was biologically inevitable and that I'd simply have to get used to weighing thirty-five pounds more. Finally I decided to see a nutritionist. This woman has taken the time to explain to me the various changes that are happening and she created a personalized diet for me, including my likes and dislikes and making sure that I get the proper amounts of vitamins and other key nutrients. After four months on this diet, I've lost fifteen pounds and am feeling much better.

Caloric needs decline by 2 percent per decade after the age of twenty. This means that the average woman in her forties (height 1.63 meters or 5 ft., 4 in., weight 54 kg or 120 lbs.) needs about 1,900 calories per day; this will dwindle to 1,800 as she approaches age fifty. Because we need fewer and fewer calories as we age, now is the time to learn about "nutrient-dense" foods and to evaluate customary intake of foods rich in vitamins A, B, and C, as well as riboflavin and folic acid. This is particularly important if alcohol is part of our routine, since alcohol inhibits the positive benefits of some vitamins and supplies "empty calories."

Vitamins A, B, and C have been found to be inadequate in the diets of many menopausal women, and these diets have probably been inadequate for some years. Vitamin B_2 (riboflavin) and folic acid (from green leafy vegetables) are related to optimum cognitive function. Because forgetfulness is a common aggravation during menopause, you can minimize the possibility by improving your diet. Your need for iron is lessened as the reproductive years draw to a close (so you can forget about *ever* learning to like liver!), but you would be wise to wean yourself away from sugar in your decaffeinated coffee and to reduce your sodium intake.

Caffeine may not keep you awake now, but many of us have belatedly discovered that it began to play a part in sleeplessness or early-morning awakening as we got older. Caffeine also blocks the absorption of calcium, which is needed for strong bones, of some B vitamins, of iron, and of Vitamin A. Caffeine may be responsible for a tendency to breast cysts and, as you get closer to the last menstrual period, often acts as a trigger for hot flashes. For diehard caffeine addicts (I was one), the potency of the product is directly related to the pain of withdrawal. If you drink a lot of coffee, tea, and/or cola drinks, giving them up may bring on a severe and prolonged headache, but this usually passes within a few days.

The good news is that there are many palatable decaffeinated beverages – including decaffeinated espresso, brewed or filtered coffees, and delicious herbal teas. Those of us who have made the switch (after years of procrastinating) try to avoid restaurants that serve packets of instant coffee with a cup of hot water and always make a point of asking for brewed decaffeinated. (Maybe eventually they'll get the message!) The rumors about decaffeinated coffees being carcinogenic (cancer causing) when treated with methylene chloride to remove the caffeine seem to be just that – rumors. The Swiss water process and the use of ethyl acetate avoid this risk, so read labels. Many restaurants also offer herbal teas, some of which are caffeine free. Ask to see the package.

Drinking black coffee (decaffeinated, that is) or clear tea (herbal, of course) requires three weeks of disciplined effort. After the taste buds are retrained, coffee or tea with sugar is like drinking syrup – fine with pancakes but too sweet as a beverage. Refined sugar contributes to the potential for high blood pressure, tends to block the benefits of some B vitamins (thiamine, riboflavin, choline, and niacin), and contributes to the incidence of nonspecific vaginitis. Because we become more and more prone to vaginal infection as we approach and pass the last menstrual period, the absence of refined sugar is a preventive against such infections, as well as against dental cavities and weight gain.

The use and overuse of salt is related to incipient high blood pressure, a condition that affects more women than men. Many women also find that it contributes to "bloat" – the unexpected and often grotesque swelling of the abdomen, which can cause extreme discomfort. Salt is an acquired taste, and most prepared foods (packaged soups and fast foods) are heavily salted to suit the taste of North Americans. Learning to do without extra salt is easier than it sounds. Lemon juice or combinations of herbs and spices are welcome substitutes, and there are many salt substitutes on the market.

The big breakthrough in nutritional research involves fat. Changes in our diet over the past half century have included enormous increases in the proportion of fats consumed as part of the so-called normal diet. It is now widely believed that a sharp reduction in the amounts and types of fat in our diet can significantly affect our predisposition to many forms of cancer, as well as to cardiovascular disease – coronary heart disease, angina, stroke, congestive heart failure, and hardening of the arteries.

Although many of us switched from butter to margarine long ago (at least at home) and reduced our consumption of eggs and fried foods in an effort to reduce dietary cholesterol, we are now told that this was either not enough or totally unnecessary (depending on whom you listen to). Many nutritionists would like us to cut down on meat (containing about 1 mg of cholesterol per gram) and eggs (containing about 250 mg each) to hold dietary cholesterol at from 250 to 300 mg per day. This can be compared with an intake of 400 mg of cholesterol per day in the average North American diet.

The information about cholesterol has been confusing because of the continuing debate about two key issues. One has to do with how cholesterol is processed by the body – how much of the cholesterol in the bloodstream is produced inside the body and how much is a result of cholesterol in the foods we eat. The other issue is the discovery that one-third to one-fifth of the population has a genetic tendency to high blood cholesterol. Until this condition was recognized, it was thought that *all* high cholesterol levels resulted from diet.

I am one of those women who has a genetic tendency to high blood cholesterol. In my case, it is due to a deficiency in choles- terol receptors – a 50 percent deficiency! I've had a dangerously high level of cholesterol for at least twenty years (260 mg/dL of blood or 6.7 mmol/L), and over these years, no amount of diet control has been able to lower the level significantly. Over the last six months, however, a new combination of drugs has low- ered it dramatically. I now feel I can look forward to a healthy level of cholesterol and even a gracious old age!

Nowadays, if a family tendency to high cholesterol levels is dis- covered (usually during routine medical checkups), potential prob- lems can be offset to some degree by scrupulous attention to diet and carefully supervised medication.

A few years ago, serum cholesterol levels (expressed either as milligrams per deciliter or millimoles per liter) were considered critical. A woman with a TC (total cholesterol) of 165 mg/dL (6.8 mmol/L) was considered to be at twice the risk of CVD compared with someone having a TC of 205 mg/dL (5.3 mmol/L). Now the concern is the ratio of HDLs to TC, the ratio of LDLs to HDLs, and the level of triglycerides.

Cholesterol circulates through the system carried by fat molecules. Some of these fats, known as HDLs (high-density lipoproteins), act to flush cholesterol and LDLs (low-density lipoproteins) out of the blood vessels. LDLs carry cholesterol into target organs, depositing it on artery walls. If LDL levels are too high, circulation clogs and clots are formed – precursors to hypertension, heart disease, and stroke. In men, the risks are associated with *both* low HDLs and high LDLs. In women, the crucial factor seems to be HDL levels, so more and more emphasis is being placed on keeping HDLs high in women at risk.

The level of HDLs (ideally, over forty) and ratio of HDLs to total cholesterol (expressed as TC/HDL) is a routine index of heart health. A ratio of 3 is excellent, meaning that HDLs constitute one-third of blood cholesterol. The ratio for the average woman is 4.5. To evaluate your own heart health, arrange for a standard blood test measuring cholesterol, lipid, and triglyceride levels. You should fast for twelve hours and avoid strenuous exercise for twenty-four hours before such a test. You need to know total blood cholesterol (TC), levels of HDLs and LDLs, *and* triglyceride levels. Total cholesterol divided by HDL, ideally, should be less than 4.0. LDLs divided by HDLs should be less than 3.0. Triglyceride levels under 200 to 250 mg/dL (2.3 to 2.8 mmol/L) are normal, while 500 mg/dL (5.6 mmol/L) is definitely too high.*

If your test results are worrisome, there's a lot of help available that will enable you to change your eating habits. The link between low fats and low heart disease and cancer rates was first noticed in countries where foods low in fat are habitually consumed. It is estimated that about 40 percent of the average diet in Canada consists

---

* Premarin at 0.625 mg daily over a period of three months will increase HDLS by an average of 16 percent, but will also increase triglyceride levels by 24 percent.

of fat, and that to ensure against a host of health risks, this should be reduced by at least 10 percent – preferably more. People who consistently adhere to a low-fat diet have been found to have reduced rates of many kinds of cancer – colorectal, prostate, breast, mouth, throat, larynx, and esophagus.

Fats in the bloodstream are hazardous not only because of the deposits they leave inside the arteries, but also because of the action of free radicals. Free radicals, which are thought to interfere with the body's defenses against cancer, are molecules that can start a chain reaction, rupturing cell membranes and crippling the body's ability to marshal cancer-preventing nutrients.

I was diagnosed as having breast cancer three years ago. Since then, I've undergone surgery and radiation therapy. It appears the cancer is now in remission. Although I'm sure the radiation has had an impact on the cancer, I wanted to tell you about the role that diet has played in my situation. Immediately after my surgery, the doctor recommended I see a dietitian. I was told to keep track of which foods I'd eaten, and how much, for two weeks. I subsequently discovered that my diet was very high in fats and that this may have had some influence on the development of cancer.

In my case, the genetic, tendency was strong (my mother died of breast cancer), but the importance of nutrition in decreasing the risks was brand-new to me. I'm not only eating better now, but, more important, I am extremely conscious of the role of diet in the (hopefully permanent) remission of this disease.

Free radicals are constantly being produced in the body, not only in response to certain foods but also as a result of pollutants in the air and other environmental factors. We cannot eliminate free radicals, but we can reduce them. Since it is believed that the metabolism of fats produces the most damaging radicals, reduction in fat intake allows the body's own defenses to mobilize and to overcome any threat posed by roaming free radicals.

Obviously, one cannot eliminate fats altogether, so it is helpful to know about various kinds of fat. Nutritionists recommend that saturated fats constitute no more than 10 percent of daily calories and that polyunsaturated (or monounsaturated) fats constitute no more than 10 percent. Saturated fats include butter, cheese, beef, veal, pork, coconut, and palm oils. Coconut and palm oil are often disguised as "vegetable oil" in prepared mixes and toppings. Polyunsaturated fats, including mayonnaise, margarine, corn oil, sunflower, and safflower oil, are fine at room temperature but, when heated, produce the free radicals thought to damage artery walls. If you want to avoid both saturated fat and the dangers of free radicals released by hot polyunsaturates, use monounsaturated fats such as olive oil or peanut oil. Or do fat-free cooking in a non-stick pan. Holding the line at 10 percent saturated plus 10 percent polyunsaturated or monounsaturated may *appear* to permit only 20 percent fats, but experts tell us that there is likely to be another hidden 10 percent consumed daily.

The dangers of red meat (as sources of both cholesterol and fat) are still very real, despite the beef industry's aggressive advertising to recapture favor. Unfortunately, the advertising doesn't respond to some basic concerns about current livestock practices. Many of us have read about the Puerto Rican children whose precocious sexual development has been traced to high levels of DES (a synthetic estrogen) fed to beef cattle. Estradiol (another form of estrogen), progesterone, and testosterone (the male hormone) are routinely fed to livestock – as are antibiotics, plastic hay, newsprint and cardboard (for roughage), and oral larvicides. Given our ignorance about the long-term consequences of these chemicals in the food chain, it is not surprising that many people choose to limit the intake of beef, pork, and veal. In other words, there is more than fat and cholesterol involved.

Vegetarians benefit from the absence of meat in their diets. Not only do vegetarians develop strong bones (they rarely suffer from osteoporosis), but organic fresh vegetables and fresh fruit also provide the kind of fiber that keeps the stomach and intestinal tract healthy. High-fiber diets appear to protect against heart disease, diverticulitis, and colon cancer, and help to avoid the kinds of problems with indigestion and constipation that are so often linked to aging.

Chicken and fish become more appealing as we age – perhaps an instance of "wisdom of the body?" Because chicken fat resides in the skin, it is easily removed, and the oilier fishes appear now to confer hidden benefits in terms of heart-protecting fatty acids. I spent years pushing fish around my plate every Friday at dinner, but now I order fish almost every time I eat out. I have found that fresh fish (and swift delivery from sea to market) makes an enormous difference – persuading me to forget an ancient grudge and to experiment with the wide range of fish available. And although I don't care to handle raw fish, it's one dish that cooks up evenly and quickly in a microwave.

It is difficult to make sudden changes in the diet, because such changes often involve new ways of cooking and new recipes to replace familiar dishes that we're used to preparing. For example, I find it virtually impossible to add up grams of fat or milligrams of calcium, not to mention caloric values. If your number memory is as poor as mine, it is helpful to check lists of foods and then to remember the *foods* that you should be eating.

I have been meeting more and more people who have seen a nutritional consultant either to lose weight or simply because they want to know more about the subject. Although the terms *dietitian* and *nutritionist* are used almost interchangeably, there *can* be a difference. Registered professional dietitians (RPDts) must meet stringent requirements: they must have completed an undergraduate or graduate degree with a program in dietetics or nutrition and have finished an approved practical program or internship. Someone who calls himself or herself a nutritionist or nutritional consultant may or may not be a dietitian, may be trained in food sciences, in biochemistry, in naturopathy – or it may just mean someone with a particular interest in health-food publications (many of which run advertisements for mail-order degrees). If you want sound advice about what you eat and how it may affect your health, make sure you know with whom you're dealing.

Until you get interested enough to formulate your own rules, here are some basic guidelines that will help you to get healthy for menopause:

- Reduce consumption of refined sugar, salt, and alcohol.
- Eliminate caffeine.
- Watch out for the tannin in tea and red wine.
- Get in the habit of drinking water; aim for six to eight glasses a day.
- Eat lots of whole-grain cereals and breads, and brown rice.
- Eat lots of fresh fruit and vegetables, preferably raw or very slightly cooked. (Store raw, cut vegetables in covered airtight containers.)
- Eat fish twice a week. Eat broiled chicken (skin removed) at least once a week.
- Explore meat substitutes (soy products like tofu, miso) in vegetarian dishes.
- Use small amounts of butter for frying; use peanut oil in wok cooking; use non-stick cookware for frying.
- Try low-fat dressings, dips, sauces (natural yogurt instead of sour cream, etc.).
- Drink four cups of skim milk or equivalent daily (containing less than one-fifth the fat content of 2 percent milk).
- Avoid bacon, cured or processed meats, or meat spreads. (Nitrites in these foods promote free radicals.)

It would take a saint to implement all these changes at once and stick to them. However, just making a few is a good start. Like all good habits, healthy eating takes practice, backsliding, and more practice.

Keeping Fit

Exercise is probably the most necessary and most overlooked prescription for a problem-free menopause. Exercise builds strong bones and tones up the cardiovascular and respiratory systems, reducing the risks of osteoporosis, arthritis, emphysema, hypertension, heart disease, and stroke.* Exercise has also been found effective in treating depression and insomnia, and in guarding against the horrors(!) of midlife weight gain. Exercise appears to increase the body's capacity to sweat easily, and the ability to sweat appears to be related to the ability to tolerate fluctuations in temperature. (A Swedish study found that women who exercise regularly and vigorously rarely have severe hot flashes.) Regular exercise is associated with a 33 percent reduction in the risk of diabetes (noninsulin-dependent diabetes mellitus). The incidence of breast, uterine, and cervical cancer is substantially reduced among women athletes. And exercise is a great way to avoid constipation and the hemorrhoids that sometimes result.

Exercise has proven beneficial for older women confined to wheelchairs; for example, regularly squeezing a tennis ball increased the strength of their arms. Unless there are valid medical reasons not to exercise, we should all be enjoying regular physical activity. Why, then, do so few of us exercise?

For too many women, exercise is anything but routine. It is something that is added to the daily (or weekly) schedule when circumstances – time, money, relationships – permit. This means that any sustained positive feelings derived from exercise are rarely experienced, or experienced for only a short time before being put aside in favor of other demands. Women over sixty who have exercised on a regular basis throughout their adult lives are rare. (Women over seventy are pearls!) I don't think it is coincidental that many nonexercisers have a difficult menopause.

When the Melpomene Institute, an organization devoted to research in women's health, conducted an informal survey of their membership to discover the reasons given for *not* being physically active, more than 90 percent of the responses involved lack of time –

---

* In a comparative study of the health status of women who had attended the same college, the women who had *not* been actively engaged in athletics were found to have 86 percent more breast cancer, and were 153 percent more likely to have developed uterine or cervical cancer, compared with their classmates who had been active in college athletics. (Frisch 1985)

either demanding jobs or overwhelming family responsibilities. But some women gave more than one reason for not undertaking regular exercise. One woman in five was afraid that she wouldn't perform well; one in six cited a lack of encouragement from others or the influence of persons who felt that she shouldn't be athletic. One in ten was influenced by others who felt that she *couldn't* be athletic. Only a small minority was held back by the perceived cost involved; far more were restrained by past or future opinions of others, whether real or anticipated. Close to 20 percent had *no* excuse for lack of physical activity.

> I want to share my experience. When I hit menopause, I immediately gained fifteen pounds. Weight gain was not unusual for me, but this time it all went to my middle, instead of clinging to my hips and thighs, as it usually does. I realized that I was dealing with a different kind of animal and that I'd better do something. I checked out a few health clubs in my area but felt like too much of an old bat to join one. I'd never been athletic and got uncomfortable merely at the thought of how I'd look in a leotard!
>
> Finally, I watched a class at the local Y and found the class for me. It's a low-impact aerobic class given in the midafternoon. I have a part-time job (mornings only), so it's great. Apart from two or three young mothers who put us all to shame, the class is made up largely of women in their forties or fifties who are afflicted with the same kind of midlife bulge as me. We laugh at ourselves and cheer each other on. Although I've lost only a few pounds, I've made some wonderful new friends and feel better than ever.

Despite the range of benefits that accrue to heart, lungs, blood vessels, bones, joints, brain, and self-image, regular exercise requires only three basic components: a warm-up, an aerobic period, and a cool-down.

The warm-up is a five- to ten-minute period of stretching, which helps to prevent injury during the more active part of the exercise. If you have ever taken part in a dance, fitness, or aerobics class, you will recognize the warm-up. But this warm-up should precede *every* kind of active exercise – before stepping onto the tennis or badminton court, or pushing off on your bicycle. If you swim, you can do stretching exercises in the shallow water before you start swimming laps. This preparation will ensure that your muscles are warm and supple. Many of the exercise tips that we learned years ago – limbering movements upon awakening, the first poses of a yoga class – fulfill this function. Vital as they are, however, they are not enough.

The core of regular physical activity is the *aerobic exercise*, a term that means the kind of strenuous exertion that carries oxygen into the system and that gets your pulse beating at a sustained rate over a period of at least twenty minutes. Aerobic exercise may include dancing, jogging, skipping, cross-country skiing, cycling, rowing, or brisk walking – any exercise that is uninterrupted and that pushes you to concentrated exertion. Most racquet sports are not particularly aerobic, but squash and handball (which involve more continuous effort) are more aerobic than tennis or badminton. (And championship levels of any racquet sport *can* be aerobic.) Swimming is aerobic only if the swimmer is going "all out" for a sustained period of time. Swimming laps may be relaxing and, to a degree, bone strengthening, but the benefits for cardiovascular fitness are debatable. Brisk walking and cycling can be both aerobic and bone building, but more beneficial to the legs than to the upper body. (Jogging and power or fitness walking require involvement of the arms as well.) Yoga and t'ai chi are not aerobic, although they increase flexibility and reduce stress.

It is the aerobic component of exercise that is directly beneficial to heart, lungs, and – if involving weight-bearing activity – to the bones. The aerobic component requires the most discipline, as one pushes oneself to breathe more efficiently (in through the nose, out through the mouth) and to perform better and longer, time after time. Because the aerobic component *is* demanding, it is recommended that every woman have a thorough physical examination before embarking on any aerobic program.

To judge whether you have had a good workout, you need to take your pulse. This can be done either in the standard way, using the wrist, or by placing your fingers under the jaw just below the ear. Count the number of beats over fifteen seconds and multiply by four. You should be aiming for a pulse rate of 220 minus your age times 0.75. (The 0.75 signifies 75 percent of maximum heart rate.) In other words if you are forty-five, you should aim for a pulse rate of 131 per minute: $220 - 45 = 175 \times 0.75 = 131$. If you are *beginning* aerobics and are over fifty, it is recommended that you look for a pulse rate of 60 percent of maximum heart rate. Using the same formula as above, this would be: $220 - 50 = 170 \times 0.60 = 102$. In time, the heart rate should be raised to around 126.

If you stop moving, the heart rate starts to plummet. If you want to monitor heart rate while exercising, slow down to a walk (don't stop), take a quick count for six seconds, and add a zero. Exceeding 80 percent of your maximum heart rate is not advisable. Once you have been doing aerobic exercise for a few weeks, you should be able to get your pulse rate up to the desired level and hold it there for twenty minutes. A lower pulse rate means you're not working hard enough.

After aerobic exercise, you need a short period of time to cool down, but be sure to wind down slowly. This is often the most overlooked aspect of an exercise program. A sudden stop is not good for the body, so walk around for a few minutes and allow your muscles to cool down. Then use a mat or folded blanket and stretch some more. Fitness instructors often add mat work to the cool-down, which may take twenty minutes or more of an hour-long class. However, the cool-down, like the warm-up, need last no more than five to ten minutes.

Experts suggest a minimum of three exercise sessions per week, with an optimum of five. Strenuous exercise every day of the week is not necessary and, in fact, may be harmful.

Time of day is up to you, but you should avoid eating just before exercise. If you have trouble getting to sleep, a brisk walk after dinner (not too close to bedtime) may alleviate the problem. If you work from nine to five, you may want to schedule your exercise for early morning, during lunch hour, or immediately after work. Investigate the kinds of facilities available in the area around your work and home. In many centers, there are free-lance fitness instructors who will lead a class if you can organize a group and find a suitable place. Low-impact exercises avoid the strain that high-impact aerobics places on knees and ankles, and are also less noisy.

If you find group exercise abhorrent, there are alternatives, but it requires dedication to get your heart rate up and keep it there. One suggestion is to get a pedometer and a Walkman (or a friend) and start a walking program. If you use a Walkman, make up your own tapes. Start your program off slowly with stretching exercises that you do at home, then begin warm-up walking, building to a brisk pace that encourages you to pump your arms; then slow down again. If you walk with a friend, arrange to meet somewhere equidistant from your homes so that you can avoid the temptation to beg off during inclement weather.

In my city, there is a group that organizes hikes every Sunday in three categories: easy, medium, and difficult. Their fee is $5 for the day. I started by going on the easy hikes, afraid I wouldn't be able to make it. But it wasn't many months before I was going on the medium hikes. I wasn't first up the hill, but I got there! Then I met the man I married and we began going on our own hikes and climbs.

My husband is a member of the Alpine Club. He introduced me to rock climbing and the use of ropes. I enjoy it, but you don't have to rock-climb in order to get exercise. A good hike up a mountain, taking small steps at a steady pace and not stopping until you have gone for an hour (and then resting) is an excellent way to get uninterrupted exercise that pushes you to concentrated exertion. And not only that – all around you is the beauty of nature and you are breathing in fresh air, not car fumes. And when you get to the top, there is the view and out comes your lunch and pot of herbal tea. What a feeling of satisfaction!

Many women feel they can get enough activity by following TV exercise programs or videotaped workouts. The problem with these is that they are either too short to bring the heart rate up for any sustained period of time or they get boring very quickly, or both. The same can be said for exercycles and skipping in place. They may be adequate for highly disciplined types who will take the time to cycle, jog, or skip in place, but most of us don't have that kind of dedication.

Women who are busy and who must cope with heavy demands at work and at home are often (understandably) reluctant to commit themselves to sessions of frantic aerobics and are more attracted to the relaxation of hatha-yoga or t'ai chi. These are marvelous adjuncts to exercise, but they don't give your heart a workout. If you are competitive by nature, you will find that the effort to keep up with a good aerobics instructor is just what you need to take a break from your problems. Because you have to concentrate on coordinating feet, arms, and breathing, you get a good forty minutes off from everyday worries.

Most of the articles and books about fitness and physical conditioning imply, and sometimes even *promise*, that exercise will restore or maintain a youthful body. This claim is misleading. You may or may not lose weight. Still, exercise has a value beyond any change in silhouette or dress size.

As we age, excess weight is deposited on different parts of the body. Through the thirties and forties, we fret about weight on the hips and thighs. As we enter the fifties, our waistlines begin to thicken and abdomens start to expand, and chest size (and often bra size) may increase. The rib cage is at its broadest between the ages of fifty-five and sixty-four. Most of these tendencies are inherited, so you probably know what to expect. Exercise may delay bodily changes due to aging, but there is no way that it can turn back the hands of the clock.

There is also a tendency to accumulate fat as we age. The body of a typical twenty-year-old woman consists of just over 25 percent fat; in the thirties and forties this increases to 33 percent and, by the fifties, to over 40 percent. Some increase in the proportion of body fat is bound to occur despite regular rigorous exercise. Even competitive women athletes (who can safely reduce body fat to no *less* than 12 percent of body weight) find that longer and harder workouts are needed to stay in shape. Physical activity will enhance a feeling of well-being for the average woman; it cannot obliterate the normal effects of age.

Nor is this all bad. As mentioned in chapter 3, women who are ten to fifteen pounds over ideal weight suffer less from severe hot flashes. (And remember that hot flashes often start a year or two before the last menstrual period.) According to the Gerontology Research Center of the U.S. National Institute on Aging, weight gain is a normal result of aging and mortality rates are *lower* for women who are slightly overweight based on standard weight and height charts.

To use their formula for calculating height and weight, divide height (in inches) by 66, multiply the result by itself, then multiply this result by your age plus 100. Let's assume you are forty-five and 5 ft. 4 in. tall: 64 (inches) divided by 66 = 0.969; 0.969 x 0.969 = 0.939; 0.939 x 145 (age plus 100) = 136 pounds. You can add or subtract nine pounds to allow for light or heavy bone structure, but this will give you a significantly higher weight than the conventional Metropolitan Life Insurance tables.

An alternative way of gauging healthy weight is the Body Mass Index (or BMI), which is mentioned in many articles about weight. This is weight in kilograms (2.2 pounds = 1 kilogram) divided by height in meters (12 inches = .3048 of a meter) squared, or kg/m^2. An easier way of using the BMI is to plot your weight on the Body Mass Index chart shown here. Find your height on line A and your present weight on line B. Draw a line through these two points and extend it to line C. If the line you draw intersects line C between 20 and 25, you are in the "normal" range – which is the range designated as producing the lowest health risks. If the index reveals a number below 20 or above 27, you are at increased risk for a number of health problems. If line C is bisected at 30 or above, you are medically "obese."

Both these newer ways of calculating weight allow for a more realistic profile and shift the emphasis away from pounds to fitness. Regular exercise may tone you and trim away inches, but may *not* trim away pounds. It will lead to cardiovascular fitness, improved muscle tone, a firmer body, and can help maintain body weight. What more do you want?

✦

Body Mass Index

6'5" •	• 320	• 37
6'4" •	• 300	• 35
6'3" •	• 280	
	• 260	• 33
6'2" •	250	
	• 240	• 31
6'1" •	230	• 30
	• 220	• 29
6' •	210	
	• 200	• 28
5'11" •	• 190	• 27
5'10" •	• 180	• 26
	• 170	• 25
5'9" •	• 160	• 24
5'8" •	• 150	• 23
		• 22
5'7" •	• 140	• 21
5'6" •	• 130	• 20
	• 120	
5'5" •		• 19
	• 110	
5'4" •		• 18
	• 100	
5'3" •		• 17
5'2" •	• 90	
5'1" •		
5' •		
A	**B**	**C**
Height (Inches)	Weight (Pounds)	BMI (In./lbs.)

Those of us who have given up smoking recognize that added weight is the price one often pays for cleaner lungs and increased life expectancy. Ex-smokers who smoked fewer than ten cigarettes a day may gain only about five pounds; those who smoked a pack or more a day may have to accept a heavier weight gain. This is not such a terrible price to pay for the health gains of *not* smoking, not to mention the benefits of once again being part of a majority!

Because so many aids are available to help one stop smoking, it seems unnecessary to preach about the evils of smoking. We know that smokers are prone to high calcium loss (resulting in brittle bones), increased risks of lung cancer, emphysema, asthma, heart disease and stroke, and earlier menopause. It is said that giving up smoking is worse than giving up heroin – I believe it! Now, having done without cigarettes for nearly twenty years, I have nothing but sympathy and support for those who are trying to kick the habit.

Many of us have abused our bodies for some time – abused in the sense of imposing additional strains by smoking, consuming too much alcohol, or perhaps relying on prescription drugs (tranquilizers or oral contraceptives) that deplete essential nutrients or that inhibit optimum brain chemistry. We abuse our bodies when we don't get regular exercise and when we forgo sensible nutrition because we are too rushed or too intent on taking care of others.

Our bodies can take a certain amount of abuse – more, if the first two decades of our lives provided a "cushion" of basic good health; less, if we have had to deal with major illness or surgery. As we look ahead to the menopausal years, we should also look for ways in which to increase stamina, endurance, and peace of mind. With luck, none of these will be jeopardized by menopause, but if they are, a well-nourished and fit body will be added insurance against the worst.

CHAPTER 9

RELATIONSHIPS AT MIDLIFE

L ife can get complicated for the menopausal woman. If her body is being buffeted by wayward hormones, she wants a predictable routine, not too much stress, and the sympathetic support of her friends and her family. Too often, the man in her life is more exasperated than sympathetic, and many women, resenting the lack of interest or concern, decide to keep their problems to themselves. But the man may also be dealing with his own demons – a nagging sense of "Is that all there is?"; a diminishing sex drive; ambivalence about impending retirement, coupled with a determination to slug it out until the best possible pension is assured.

The menopausal mother may be dealing as well with inconsiderate teenagers (are there any other kind?) or with young adults who leave home, only to return weeks or months later, adding yet one more element of unpredictability to her life. Or she may find that her home is suddenly empty. There may be aging parents who need her to run errands, to do shopping, to accompany them to the doctor. And today, on top of all this, she is likely to be holding down a full-time job.

If a woman is feeling well, these various demands can sometimes be juggled quite successfully. If she is not feeling well, the pressure can be overwhelming. It helps to know that it is happening to others. It helps to discuss the situation with friends, because by talking it over you can often sort out which demands on your time should take priority and why. Remember, this too shall pass.

Female Friendships

It's unfortunate that many of us have to wait until our forties or fifties to cherish the commonsense advice and support that we receive from our female friends. Our single friends have learned to value their married women friends, and many of the newly divorced or widowed quickly relearn the value of friends, but too many married women make room for female friendships only in the spaces not occupied by husbands and children. I'm sorry that I waited so long to find time for my friends – meeting for dinner, meeting for a weekend at a country inn, making impromptu long-distance calls just to keep in touch. Once upon a time, those of us without dates on a Friday or Saturday night would congregate for an evening of talk about life, love, and the pursuit of happiness. For many of us, that was the last real taste of woman-to-woman intimacy until the kitchen coffee klatch, where toddlers bounced against us as we chatted. Now we are rediscovering friendship as we experienced it in our late teens and early twenties. And it is good. We wonder why it ever stopped. Finances got in the way, that's true, but the real obstacle was our own well-learned ethic: The man takes precedence. Being married and staying married pushed same-sex friendships aside. It's interesting to trace this ethic, this notion of woman as eternal competitor for the man. Hardly an attitude that fosters cordial woman-to-woman relationships.

Historically, women have found support, sympathy, and understanding from other women. Their common experience fostered a closeness quite different from the primarily economic ties to men. Written documents of earlier centuries reveal strong bonds uniting female relatives and friends, with common interests in domestic matters, the hazards of pregnancy and childbirth, and the aching suspense of nursing family members through illness. Because women's interests were sharply divided from men's, each sex was more likely to discuss matters of common interest with same-sex friends.

Also, there were more single women in those days. Widows and spinsters lived with the family, providing respite from child care for the mother and support for one another. This must have been helpful to mothers, not only in practical ways, but as a constant reminder that there was more to life than children and husbands. We need that kind of reminding even more today, because those of us who are wives and mothers are often too preoccupied with the effect of menopause on family members. We ignore our single friends, whose experience of menopause is different but no less valid. We should be learning from one another.

Marriage has assumed more importance in this century, and since the culture dictated that a married woman had more status than a single woman, women began to view one another as competitors for a scarce resource. Social life marched two-by-two and "singles" were made to feel like third thumbs.

> When I ran my first Midlife Workshop for Women, the energy generated by women sharing their life experiences could have illuminated the room. Throughout the workshop, women felt an intense closeness and bonding with each other and kept asking, "How come we've been so separated from each other all these years? Why have we each felt so isolated?"
>
> Finally, someone said it: "Our men kept us apart. We were so afraid of losing our men to other women that we cut back on our female friendships!"

Women also looked for an ideal marriage relationship – a caring, supportive, understanding partner in whom to confide, on whom to rely, with whom to discuss and share everything. Very few marriages fulfill this ideal, and the high rates of divorce and separation during the past few decades are testimony to the disillusionment inherent in such an unrealistic expectation. But the majority of marriages endure, and because the illusion of an ideal marriage must be perpetuated, many married women continue to turn aside opportunities for friendship. By limiting their intimate friendships to one heterosexual relationship, such women are inviting spiritual anorexia – pointlessly starving themselves of friends.

Men often define a friend as someone to do things with. Women tend to define a friend as someone to talk to, to share feelings with. Women are more likely to recognize the connectedness of relationships; their decisions and actions take into account the effect on others, regardless of the absolute "right" or "wrong" of the situation. Where men see a hierarchy – "Who was in charge?" "Is that part of his job?" – women see a network – "Did everyone help out?" "How did she feel?" For men, power and control take precedence; friendship must bow to rules that separate employee from employer, member from nonmember. Women are more likely to overlook status differences where mutual interests are recognized.

Given these different ways of viewing the world, it is easier to understand why women are receptive to the idea of intimate friendship and so lost without it, and why men, although open to the idea of friendship *in principle*, will often forgo it for the sake of a job, a title, the rules, or the team. What is hard to understand is female complicity in the "put-down" of women-only social situations. Women who fail to recognize the deep-seated male envy of female friendships may be lured into trivializing something that is important to them. Many women who once gained support and sympathy in hastily convened kitchen meetings now attend more formal business meetings – to find that, aside from the constant interruption of children, more problems were solved in those informal get-togethers than are solved by most highly organized committees.

No one should be without a friend. There are all sorts of opportunities at work (paid or volunteer), in educational or recreational settings, in social situations linked to work or club membership. Why, given all these opportunities, do some women still feel friendless? Part of it may be the low level of self-esteem that follows from being housebound. Some of it is sheer lack of experience in nurturing friendship. Some of it comes from a misplaced reticence about "personal matters."

I learned very early in life that I couldn't trust my friends. Being a very sensitive child, it went pretty deep when I had been betrayed. Already a loner and middle child, it didn't take much for me to sort of abandon the human race and live a rather lonely life for many years. When I would occasionally long for a friend, of course there was nobody there.

In recent years, I have stretched out my hand more and more (if you want a friend, you have to be a friend), but it is hard work for me. A few times when I have reached out to a person with whom I felt I had something in common, I was rejected. I blamed it all on myself but have since learned that I shouldn't. (I've always been hard on myself.) Maybe I was just trying too hard. I envy those who have cultivated true friendships, but haven't given up hope yet of acquiring the same for me.

It is difficult to become intimate with a woman who avoids self-disclosure. It is impossible to complain about one's own husband (inconsiderate lout!) to a woman who admits no flaw in her own, to express outrage about one's children (ungrateful wretches!) to a woman who appears to have perfect offspring, to mutter about the ceaseless demands of an aging parent to a woman who is a Florence Nightingale. Perhaps such women feel that to admit to a problem would be to lower themselves in the eyes of others. Frankly, I find such attitudes a barrier to friendship. How wonderful to have a woman friend who makes no judgment calls, who allows you to unload all the anger, disappointment, and spite, and who is never surprised to find that after all the anguish, you've forgiven and forgotten by the following day.

The female definition of friendship is percolating into the business world. As women break into higher ranks of management, customs of informal socializing on the job are not only being tolerated, but are being encouraged because they contribute to higher productivity and morale. Seminars run by women bring groups of business people together to talk about attitudes or habits that are impediments to personal or professional progress. These seminars are not promoted as teaching "feminine" skills, but that is precisely what is going on.

For many of us, female friendships grow sweeter as the years go by. Many of us have more time to spend with friends, to linger over a glass of wine, to visit for weekends, to meet for all-day shopping binges, or to spend a few days enjoying shared interests. This is one of the bonuses of menopause. The pain and the puzzlement can be shared with our women friends. Menopause gives us an opportunity to strengthen old friendships or to forge new ones – friendships that will stand us in good stead in the years to come when many of the men in our lives will have passed on.

Women who have chosen to remain single can teach us the value of friendship. Women without partners, whether through death or divorce, find that female friends provide a safety net, a web of caring to keep them from hitting bottom. Our friends are companions in new adventures, sounding boards as we embark on a new stage of life. They share a range of experience that is unique to women.

Long-Term Relationships

One evening after dinner, during my fifty-first year, I found myself pulling off my wedding ring and hurling it at my husband while I shrieked my intention of seeing a divorce lawyer. What had come over me? Too much wine, for one thing, and a great deal of emotional confusion. We didn't speak for the rest of that evening, but we did climb into the same bed (every other bed being occupied that night). I woke up at two a.m., wondering whether I had finally lost my grip, and went downstairs to sit and think. Fortunately, my husband noticed my absence and came down to talk. We had had many, many emotional scenes in our twenty-seven years of marriage but we had *never* mentioned divorce before. And I had been the one to bring it up! I couldn't understand what was happening to us.

In successful long-term relationships, there is an unspoken agreement. When *he* is feeling dejected and discouraged, *she* will be upbeat and optimistic. When *she* is feeling worn-out and useless, *he* will tell her she's one in a million. Marriage consists, in large part, of cheering each other up.

Then along comes menopause and midlife. Frequently, both partners are consumed with their individual and very real problems, and the unspoken agreement goes out the window. At least, that's my best guess at what happens.

Menopause often comes at a time when the husband is making a last-ditch effort to secure his place at work. The years just before retirement are the years that dictate the dollar value of his pension. They are also years when maintaining energy and dedication to the job may become more and more difficult. So the man is often under strain.

If there are adolescent children in the house, this adds to the tension. Even the best-behaved teenager knows how to manipulate parents to get his or her way, and that manipulation often creates a divisive atmosphere. One parent views the other as either too lax or too strict. More havoc is caused by teenagers whose styles of dress, tastes in music, attitudes toward education or money (or both) become, implicitly or explicitly, threats to parental values. Such challenges to authority often arise at a time when Father is dealing with his private insecurities and Mother is not feeling up to assuming her usual role of mediator.

Where the children are older and away from the house, there are other strains. Sometimes men are winding down their jobs just as their wives, newly liberated from domestic responsibilities, are gearing up. Many women in their late forties or early fifties bravely return to school or to the work force – or both – with the heady intention of now doing what *they* want to do. Women who have always been in the work force may find renewed energy for their jobs as household chores take a backseat. The husband who has been looking forward to spending more time with his wife (now that the children are gone) may find that she is rarely there. She is wrapped up in new and exciting interests that he cannot or will not share.

Then there is the effect of menopause itself. It often brings on mood swings – emotional ups-and-downs that are difficult for both the woman and her husband to understand or contend with. There is something eerily reminiscent of adolescent emotionality in the yo-yo action of menopausal moods. But this is not the whole story. It seems to me that there has been too much focus on the mood swings of the menopausal woman and too little attention paid to the male half of the equation.

It is *assumed* that the woman is being difficult during menopause, and she may be. But many men continue to think of themselves as the sweet, good-tempered souls they were at age twenty-five or thirty. They forget about the invisible but unavoidable transfer of attitudes from work to home. If they have achieved any sort of authority on the job, that authority may also be exerted at home. The habits acquired when commanding others, when delegating chores, when minimizing complaints among subordinates, when problem solving, may get in the way of the ability to listen, to sympathize, and to learn. This may be even more true of the man who has not been as successful as he had hoped. His need for admiration and respect may get in the way of the intimacy that his wife had expected from long-term marriage.

One of the greatest threats to good marriage at midlife is the sense of vulnerability that many women feel. When they look at their husbands, they see people who are trudging through life at a steady pace, aging slowly but often attractively, looking more prosperous and more confident than ever. In our society, the media present us with images of successful middle-aged men every day – in advertisements, in the news, in business appointments, in TV shows. The graying, slightly corpulent middle-aged man often achieves an air of distinction denied to him at a younger age. And why *shouldn't* he look distinguished? Heaven knows, he's worked hard enough for it!

Then we look at ourselves. We see signs of aging (thickened waist, graying hair, aching joints) that arrive too quickly to be properly assimilated. Positive role models are scarce. There are middle-aged women in show business who continue to look thirty-five, and a few women in public life who radiate confidence and competence.

But it is hard to find a woman to emulate, an image to aim for. In a society that celebrates youth, we judge ourselves as second rate – physical well-being unpredictable, confidence sagging. It's hard to discuss this with a husband. Why point out to him how fat you're getting if he hasn't noticed? Why tell him how miserable you're feeling when you know (and he knows) that there isn't any *reason* for you to feel so unsure of yourself? How many husbands have exasperatedly terminated a conversation with "Why not see a doctor?" How many wives have given up trying to make him understand?

> For many years, when the kids were small, my husband often went to bed for a nap right after supper. By the time he got up again, it was bedtime for the children. On days he didn't nap, there was a meeting, or a course to go to, or a workout at the local YMCA. As a full-time homemaker, I cannot tell you how disappointed, frustrated, and angry I was when I didn't get the support I thought I needed – after having already spent all day alone with the little ones.
>
> I felt I just *had* to get involved in the community in order to keep my sanity. Before long, I was into various things that I very much enjoy but that keep me away from home some evenings. Since I'm still a full-time homemaker, with the kids at school and hardly anybody to talk to during the day, my contacts with these people in the evenings are my lifesavers. These groups have – in the absence of any relatives in North America – become my support system.
>
> But now my husband is going through his own "change of life" as well. He demands more time, attention, ego stroking, etc., and almost resents it when I'm out, sometimes a few evenings in a row. He stays home most evenings since he is feeling depressed and hasn't much energy. Doesn't that sound familiar? Now and then he says, "I don't seem to be too high on your list," or "Do I have to make an appointment with you?"
>
> Not only have I got nothing to spare right now in the way of care giving, but I also keep asking myself, "Where

was *he* when I needed *him?*" Besides, I feel I have to have my own needs met for a change before I can be an effective care giver again.

Many of us had already learned to "keep a cap on it" during the few days prior to our monthly menstrual periods. At "that time of the month," we could easily turn a minor skirmish into a full-scale war, so we learned (the hard way) to grit our teeth and keep quiet. It seems to me that menopause is often a prolonged premenstrual period. Instead of keeping a cap on it for two or three days, we may have to keep mum for two or three years. This is not easy to do, and we all forget our good intentions and blurt out hurtful criticisms now and then, but at least we're trying. And we're trying because we have a profound confidence in the viability – and durability – of the relationship.

It takes years to develop that kind of confidence: to know, at a gut level, that this is someone you want to spend your old age with, God willing. I know many women who don't feel that way. Some have decided to call it quits: the only common interest that had endured was the children. Others have decided to hang in: they are realists and recognize that they will never achieve the standard of living alone that they have become accustomed to as wives. I don't think men realize just how many women, smiling and compliant as they may appear, are living with these kinds of decisions.

I also know many women who have a great deal more in common with their husbands than they are willing to acknowledge. A divorced friend of mine refers to her ex-husband as her "history" – as much a part of her, after more than twenty-five years of marriage, as part of her own body. She does not regret her decision to divorce, but it took the divorce to make her recognize this shared past. Another friend made a different decision. After living apart from her husband for almost two years, she swallowed her pride and decided to go back. They have no more in common than they had when she left, but they both appreciate each other more because of the separation. As this friend said, "Any habit is hard to break, and we had the habit of living together." Another friend is muddling through, as she says, by "reviving some of the customs of early married life." By this, she means being conscientiously *nice* – complimenting her husband when he does or says something positive, being more polite than usual, and, in general, being as considerate as she was at the beginning of married life. Her hope is that the marriage will evolve, as it did once before, into a comfortable relationship.

There are a lot of marriages that exist in the space between commitment (contented or working at it) and hostility (veiled or open). Some are jeopardized by sexual matters: wives who find sexual desire absent after surgery or who can no longer experience orgasm as they once did, husbands who disguise their own faltering sex drive by blaming their partners. Some relationships are fraught with the fear of disappointing, haunted by one partner's sense of never quite reaching the promise implied so many years ago. Some couples are so busy looking at the *little* differences that they never stop to recognize large areas of their lives that offer mutual interest and delight. These are the marriages that could be enriched by a few sessions with a qualified marriage counselor.

The challenges and rigors of menopause will never be understood by a man. Expecting much more than tolerance and forbearance may be expecting too much. Marriage at midlife may not be too different from marriage at any other time – great, rotten, or somewhere in between – but it may be all of these things within the span of one day. This may be a time to cherish what you've got, to put it on "hold" as best you can, and to promise yourself to be good to him when you're feeling better.

Male Menopause

For some time now I have felt that I, as well as my wife, am going through some bodily change. I feel on top of the world one day and just the opposite the next. I also don't have that *joie de vivre* that I was used to. What really concerns me is my sex drive, which at times just disappears. I am used to having a normal male sex drive and enjoy it very much; to suddenly find it evaporate for no reason is very hard to handle.

This letter conveys the essence of the so-called male menopause – the absence of sex drive. Actually, there is no such thing as "menopause" for the male, because menopause requires a monthly menstrual period, but the term has been freely borrowed to describe problems that sometimes bother midlife males – the absence of sexual desire and/or the inability to sustain an erection. Even when other symptoms are mentioned, these two assume paramount importance.

Male menopause is not the same thing as *midlife crisis* – a term that is applied mainly to men between forty and fifty. This age rarely marks the real midpoint of a man's life, but it assumes the earmarks of "crisis" because the fortieth year has assumed great significance for men in Western society. In Europe, the syndrome (if indeed it exists) is known as *andropause* and is receiving more and more attention from both social scientists and researchers.

Because the average adult male experiences a lengthy and very gradual reduction in the production of androgens, particularly testosterone, he is less likely to suffer from the kind of abrupt changes experienced by the average female at menopause. It seems likely, however, that *some* men (no one knows exactly how many) may be prone to sudden drops in hormone levels at midlife. The statistic that is frequently quoted is 15 percent, but it is not substantiated, and little or no attention is paid to other factors that might significantly affect testosterone levels (e.g., smoking, alcohol intake, and effects of medications).

Hormone levels are also influenced by stress. Many men in their late forties and early fifties are dealing with job-related tension – tension stemming from unrelenting effort, from pressure, from frustration, from apprehension, or from boredom and monotony. The tension may be compounded at home, particularly when there are adolescent children. The man may be consuming too much food and too much alcohol. He may be experiencing new and annoying infirmities – a sore back, bursitis, inflamed or enlarged prostate. Any combination of these symptoms could lead to *secondary* testicular failure, or the temporary inability to produce adequate amounts of testosterone. This leads directly to loss of sexual desire.

Sexual performance is so intricately tied to a man's self-image that emotion often supplants reason. For many men, it is not so much the reduction in sex drive that is threatening, but the loss of what is seen as "manhood." To avoid dealing with the problem, he finds excuses. He may work late and come home exhausted; he may stay up to watch late-night television, allowing his wife to get to sleep first; he may start arguments so he can go to bed mad. In some cases, the wife may be held responsible for his inability to "turn on" – she is not inviting, or enticing, or aggressive, or compliant, or available enough.

The stress of feeling inadequate can lead to impotence, the inability to sustain an erection. Again, this type of impotence is considered secondary because there is no functional block to potency. (One of the ways to determine if impotence is primary or secondary is to look at the man's capacity for erection when waking up in the morning or during dream sleep. If he can have an erection at these times, then impotence is considered secondary.)

Once upon a time, urologists were intent on discriminating between primary and secondary testicular failure. Now they have Viagra. Most will just assume that the impotence is secondary, that it is resulting from stress, and hand out a prescription.

However, should a man be suffering from primary testicular failure, it is not only his potency as a sex partner that suffers. Deficiencies in testosterone may be responsible for declining musculature, increased body fat, and thinner bones – and may also influence mood. However, testosterone therapy is a tricky business. Hormone levels are measured in picograms or nanograms – one trillionth or one billionth of a gram. Too much testosterone may have an impact on heart function (as does Viagra if it interacts with some heart medications). Because the difference between 'enough' and 'too much' added testosterone is difficult to establish, there is an understandable reluctance to do too much experimenting.

If it is felt that impotence is due to primary testicular failure, tests will be ordered to measure testosterone and gonadotropin levels. (Just as women secrete small amounts of testosterone, men secrete small amounts of FSH, LH – and estrogen!) The tests are not always accurate, however. As we know from female physiology, very small variations in hormone levels can produce remarkable effects. Unless the tests demonstrate a clear physical malfunction, most doctors will assume the impotence is *secondary testicular deficiency* resulting from stress.

In 1989, Dr. John McKinlay, epidemiologist and principal investigator for the Massachusetts Male Aging Study, reacted to the prospect of treating male menopause:

> I don't believe in the male midlife crisis. But even though, from my perspective, there is no epidemiological, physiological, or clinical evidence for such a syndrome, I think by the year 2000 the syndrome will exist. There's a very strong interest in treating aging men for a profit just as there is for menopausal women.

Dr. McKinlay's prophecy has certainly come true. I have no doubt that Viagra has brought a measure of sexual satisfaction to many men and their partners since its introduction. What I remember vividly, however, are the comments of gynecologists at a North American Menopause Society meeting in the late 90's. They spoke about the repercussions of Viagra – the increasing numbers of late middle-aged women who opted for estrogen to "keep their vaginas young" and the increased demand for vaginal creams and lubricants. I gather that some of their 60- and 70-year-old female patients were not entirely pleased with their newly-vigorous husbands!

Rather than moving gently and contentedly into the companionship of old age, the over-fifties are supporting a whole new industry!

The Empty Nest

According to the *Second Barnard Dictionary of New English*, the *empty nest syndrome* is a "form of depression supposedly common among women whose children have grown up and left home." The term was first used in a book published in 1952 but became common currency in the mid-1960's. The operative phrase is "supposedly common." For every woman suffering from empty nest syndrome, there are many others who feel guilty because they're so glad or relieved to have the children leave. The phrase is perpetuated not by women, but by advertisers who push medication or new furniture as a cure for the temporary lull between stages of a woman's life.

The empty nest conjures up a picture of a woman alone in a house designed and furnished for a family. How applicable is this to women today? Not all women live in houses; not all are mothers with grown children; very few women spend their days at home. It assumes that women have neither the foresight nor the adaptability to take up new interests or activities as the children become more independent. It also assumes that the children have left for good.

Most of the women I have heard from are not at all depressed by an empty nest. They find their ordered lives, their neater rooms, their freedom to come and go a welcome change. Many also think of themselves as "unnatural mothers," not realizing that all available research findings agree that there is a very welcome increase in satisfaction with life after the departure of the last child – less concern about the children, more activities with husband and/or friends, and increased marital happiness.

> I can really relate to others who are saying goodbye to their last child. Our youngest, who is now twenty-three, has just moved out for the last time. He has come home several times but we have now told him that this time he is on his own. We are hoping it will work out, since he is now sharing a home with his sister. Guilt? None.
> It is great to know you can cook for two and only two will show up, and that there are times you can come home

to a tidy and empty house. I really enjoy being able to go to bed at my early hour and have the house quiet enough to sleep. My husband works shifts, so I'm often the only one home and I love it!

This is not to say that we don't experience strong feelings as the children leave. The "launching" of the last child marks the end of a period in our lives and forces us to acknowledge the passing of time. I remember crying when my eldest started first grade (I was expecting my fourth child at the time!) and when I was folding away the baby clothes after the fifth and last had outgrown them. Both events marked an end and a beginning, which is why I cried. But there was no real yearning to go back. And so it is for most women when the last child leaves.

The real emptiness that many of us dread derives from aspects of motherhood that are rarely discussed: the loss of both intimacy and control. Motherhood involves enormous power – a power that we acknowledge mostly in its negative form as child abuse, but power nonetheless. With the departure of the children, many women lose a sense of power and purpose that is denied them in any other sphere. This loss is real and difficult to replace.

I believe I have a classic case of empty nest. I have five children, and the youngest, now twenty-four, recently moved out on her own. For the last four or five years, I've been feeling guilty about actually wanting her to leave. My marriage has never been the greatest, and I always hoped that extended periods of time alone would help the relationship between me and my husband. Unfortunately, I find myself feeling more alone than ever.

My husband has never been a good communicator and he continues to shut me out of his life. My problem is one of conflicting emotions. On the one hand, I feel relieved that my children are gone, but I also feel enormous guilt, because I feel I may have pushed or prodded them out of the house. Now that they're gone, I miss the closeness and involvement in their daily lives, something I never get from my husband.

The departure of the children creates a lull, and many of us find ourselves off kilter as we grope for new ways to feel a sense of accomplishment. But the lull is temporary. Most of us can turn to friends, to work – volunteer or paid – to a husband, or to a lover to take up the slack.

A more common concern than empty nest, according to my correspondents, is the child who leaves, returns, and leaves again. Many women feel guilty that they don't miss their children more after they've left. Many feel guiltier still when the return of the child doesn't lift the heart, or lifts it for only a day or two! And yet, in these days of mounting tuition fees and escalating rents, many young adults *must* move home if they want to continue their education or get a leg up in the job market. And who is going to turf them out?

A researcher in England investigated parents' feelings about the empty nest. She found that mothers and fathers felt very differently about the departure of a child, depending on the age of the child, where the child was going, the personality of the child, and the relationship with the parent or parents. This study highlights the complexity of a situation that has been simplistically exploited by the media. Women who talk to other women recognize that each situation – like each child – is unique, that the term *empty nest* suggests much but describes very little.

The Sandwich Generation

Over past years, the phrase *sandwich generation* has become generally accepted as a way of describing midlife women and men who are required to deal, at the same time, with the needs of both the older generation and the younger one – their parents and their children. More and more middle-aged women are experiencing the squeeze of the sandwich. Elaine Brody calls them "women in the middle," caught between the needs of aging parents and the demands of the children (and often grandchildren). Many are also caught between seething resentment and bouts of self-imposed guilt.

Our parents can expect to live longer these days. This is not necessarily a result of improved medical care (although this does play a
part). Better education has led to improved hygiene and nutrition.
There are also *more* old people relative to the population as a whole.
As families have become smaller and as immigration has slowed, we
have seen a steady increase in the proportion of elderly in our society. Those over sixty-five now constitute 12.6 percent of the population; in only a few years, they will make up 15 percent. The aged are
becoming more visible simply because there are more of them.

This has many effects. When the aged constitute a small proportion of the population, they are highly prized. They are the repositories of the oral history of a people, the witnesses to "the way we
were." The child with a grandparent is special and is envied. As the
aged population increases, veneration and respect for the individual
yield to concern for and interest in the many. The study of all aspects
of aging (gerontology) and the care of the aging (geriatrics) attract
more interest and more tax dollars. Today researchers in the field no
longer talk about the "old," but about the "young-old" (aged fifty-
five to seventy-five) and the "old-old" (aged seventy-five upward).
The young-old are often the chief caretakers of the old-old.

One of the great ironies of the generation of women now dealing with menopause is that, after thirty years of hard work, they
often find themselves better off than both their parents *and* their
children. Most of us had expected to do better than our parents
and many of us did. But this prospect has faded for our children,
who form part of the first generation to be denied a standard of living higher than that of their parents. This means that many of us
are caught between the demands of a younger generation with
extended dependency needs and an older generation too proud to
ask for help.

Many of us are forced to acquire new skills. As parents, we must
adopt a tactful and neutral silence when our grown children make
silly mistakes – the kind of mistakes that *we* made when well out of
the sight and sound of Mom and Dad. At the same time, we are
required to muster diplomatic skills in order to intervene in the best
interests of parents. For the sandwich generation, the problem is how

to "be there" for children and for parents – to help out when needed and to stand aside when appropriate. It is normal and natural to
resent the encroachment on one's time. It is also normal and natural
to feel apprehension at the prospect of years of caregiving to parents,
particularly when the caregiving to children must go on.

> I feel like I am in a double-decker sandwich. I am, after
> twenty-five years of marriage, a single parent. I have a
> daughter twenty-two, and a son twenty, still living with me.
> I love them both dearly. I have been alone with them now
> for five years. They are adults, but because they are living
> with me, they still demand a great deal of my time, directly
> or indirectly. They contribute financially, but emotionally,
> when you get three very strong-willed adults, there are
> bound to be waves from time to time.
>   Then there is my seventy-year-old mother, who is not
> well and who is unable to do much for herself. I do her
> errands and many other things. At first, I was foolishly run-
> ning myself off my feet, and found this very draining. I
> finally woke up to the realization that my mother, who had
> never worked out of the home, just did not realize the
> demands she was making on me. I am employed full-time
> and simply had to establish some priorities. Once she got
> to know when I would be coming over, that this would be
> regular and that she could count on it, there was no problem.
>   I don't think we should feel guilty if we put restrictions
> on our time. I think that what makes it difficult for the
> elderly is the uncertainty of their lives. Once they can rely
> on a regular routine (of visits, shopping, etc.), it is easier
> to cope.

Women reputed to be good managers can never rest on their lau-
rels. The women who "cope" are the women who spring to mind
when there is an unexpected need for someone to manage a crisis.
Many events conspire to designate this "woman in the middle" – traditional attitudes about the roles and "innate" capabilities of women,

experience with childhood crises, attention and sensitivity to family relationships. It is not justice that seeks her out, but rather her demonstrated ability to deal with one more family crisis.

This woman may still be the major caregiver for the children – those still at home and those who return. Chances are that she has always taken care of the weekly grocery shopping, the nightly dinner, the clean sheets, and the "pick-it-up-and-put-it-away." Women seem to be stuck with this role. And even though many of us work outside the home, we are married to men who take it for granted that men's work is more important than women's, and that wives are biologically programmed to take care of the needs and niceties of "family" – extending invitations, remembering birthdays, sending gifts, offering services. We may chafe at this particular role now (although it may have been a shared expectation twenty years ago), but by fulfilling it, we are perpetuating it.

The "woman in the middle" recognizes herself. She knows, as do her brothers, sisters, and in-laws, that when the time comes, she will be the one who is called upon. The story of the family where brothers and sisters spend equal amounts of time and effort amicably caring for aging parents must be a fairy tale. (Just like the one where other members of the family *don't* tell you what to do about the adult children still underfoot!)

Women feel guilty about resenting adult children and they feel guilty about resenting the demands of aging parents. One expert on aging says that,

> ... the most dominant and pervasive issue regarding intergenerational relationships is the subject of guilt. Often the adult offspring feel responsible for the general well-being of parents, [although they] frequently cannot improve their parents' general satisfaction with life. (Ragan 1979)

This issue of guilt is important, because it is guilt that leads dutiful daughters to say, "They took care of me as a child. It is my turn to take care of them now." But taking care of a child is done with the expectation that the child will become more independent and more self-sufficient. This kind of expectation is *not* realistic in relation to aging parents.

What kinds of expectations *are* realistic? First of all, it may be *very* realistic to anticipate that you will do most of the worrying and most of the work. Sons tend to become caregivers only when they have no sisters, and even then are more likely to call on their wives for "hands-on" help when dealing with their own parents. Sons may be called upon for financial advice and for physical tasks (lifting and carrying), but the women are almost always the primary caregivers. And the woman is typically a married, adult daughter (or daughter-in-law), a mother, and often a grandmother.

> Last week, Mom phoned every night, feeling terrible. I'd already taken time off (no pay) to take her to see two doctors and I had no car for two days. I finally phoned my brother and said, "You take Mom to the doctor's." "But, but ... I'm busy," etc., etc. Finally I said, "You do it!" And he did. Hooray for persistence.
>
> We are so used to being members of a generation where the woman does everything, it's hard to stop and say, "Excuse me, how about thinking about me?" We should get someone to shoulder it, but that will never change for us.
>
> After Mom's second fall and hospitalization, I pulled over to the side of the road on the way home and had a good cry. I'm stressed, but I can handle it. I have my man to complain to, my good friends, my workmates, and my daughters. Because I'm relating this situation to my own aging, I'm learning. The guilt never goes, but I will myself through it, and God gives me patience and comfort to understand and try to help. I might be in my mother's place soon and I'm thankful that I have two daughters who will care for me.

It is *not* realistic to expect that gratitude for services rendered will smooth out rocky relations between the generations. If there is any kind of personality clash, it is likely to get worse, not better, as time goes on. Parents are always parents and they continue to feel and behave in parental ways. They are likely to stay the same, only more so, and their criticism or praise continues to have enormous influence on us, whether positive or negative. If they have no economic clout to wield, parents can still motivate us through flattery, gratitude, or guilt.

Nor is it realistic to expect that being surrounded by family will erase the void that the aged feel when continually confronted by the death of friends. Aging parents need friends. Family members, no matter how well intentioned, cannot substitute for the sense of well-being provided by friendship and common interests. You can help your aging parents to feel more comfortable, but you may not be able to change their general level of satisfaction with life.

It may be wise to examine your intentions, however honorable, and your motivation in assuming care of aging parents. Remind yourself that it is possible not to love someone and still care for him or her. Even if you feel genuine love for an aging parent, there will be times when you find it hard to like this person. Whether motivated by love, liking, duty, guilt, or a constantly changing mixture of all of these, there will be times when you feel squeezed beyond recognition.

When parents feel that they can no longer cope with a young adult child who is not working, seems unable to find a job, is doing poorly at school, is planning to return home, appears unable to cope on his/her own, etc., most will seek help. They turn to the resources that their tax dollars put in place. Academic advisers and trained counselors are available in high schools, colleges, and universities. They can tap into job retraining schemes, government bursaries, student-loan plans, employment opportunities, or psychological services. If there is genuine conflict over goals set by you, your husband, or your adult child, then family counseling may be recommended. Most parents are more likely to take advantage of such services, once they know about them, because it is for the child's ultimate benefit.

Unfortunately, many of us do not carry this attitude through when dealing with aging parents. Guilt gets in the way and we view the use of community resources as an abandonment of responsibility. We consider it a personal failure if we are unable to fulfill the needs of our parents, although this is as unrealistic as expecting to fulfill *all* the needs of our children, needs that cannot be foreseen or whose satisfaction is beyond our expertise.

Ideally, provision of care for aging family members should take into account the opinions of the parent or parents. Even when aging parents deny the encroaching limitations of old age – "I'm fine, dear. Don't worry about me!" – this is no reason to postpone planning for the future. At the very least, you can explore the facilities available in the community and plan accordingly. If your parent willingly participates in the discussion, so much the better.

Depending on such factors as income, time commitments, and geographical location, what responsibilities will be undertaken by other family members? What are your parents' financial resources, now and in the years to come? What kinds of alternative living arrangements might be acceptable to them, and what kinds of waiting lists do the "approved" facilities have? What kinds of community resources are available to help your parent(s) stay in their own home?

If a parent is seeing the doctor frequently, you may wish to find out if a geriatric screening program is available. This will permit a thorough and comprehensive examination without having to make appointments with a number of specialists. The resulting report will give you and your parent(s) a clear idea of their health status and may help to allay fears and/or lead to more constructive planning for the future.

Become familiar with the resources available in your parents' community – integrated homemaking care (cleaning and shopping services), Meals on Wheels, telephone checks, special medical alarms (easily tripped to elicit a return call and/or calls to a doctor, neighbor, nearby relative, or ambulance service), escort or transportation services, and help with home maintenance. You may be able to arrange for a public-health nurse, podiatrist, or hairstylist to visit. (Care of the hair gets more difficult for women as they age, and care of the feet is particularly important if older people are to remain mobile and healthy.)

If you feel that a parent should not be left alone, you may be able to find sitting services. Some old-age homes also offer "respite care" – short-term accommodation (from a few days to a few weeks) in a supervised setting so that the caregivers can have a weekend off or a vacation. It is wise to familiarize yourself with all these services before you have to call on them.

Sometimes all the resources in the world cannot relieve the psychological stress of being responsible for family members. More and more community organizations are organizing support groups for caretakers of the aging. These groups may not be able to *change* the situation, but they can offer the opportunity to meet with others in the same situation, to air grievances, anxieties, guilt feelings, and to ventilate the anger that accumulates. It may also help you to deal with the frustration at your inability to "make it all go away," to make things better for your parent(s) – an inability that we may recognize intellectually but that is difficult to accept emotionally.

The "woman in the middle" lives between the stress of competing "guilts." Braced for the accusation that she has never been as good a mother as she had intended to be, she accuses herself of not being the loving and dutiful daughter that her parents deserve. The myth of the "good mother," coupled with the myth of the "good daughter," is powerful indeed. Women are tough meat in the sandwich.

CHAPTER 10

AGING AND
APPEARANCE

*Aging is much more a social judgment than a biological eventuality.
Far more extensive than the hard sense of loss suffered during
menopause ... is the depression about aging, which may or may
not be set off by any real event in a woman's life ...*

— Susan Sontag, "The Double Standard of Aging"

Despite all the protestations (and reassurances) that
menopause and middle age are two separate and
separable events, the lived experience of women fuses them.
Menopause means growing older, becoming invisible, losing one's
power and one's credibility. Our higher intellectual functions may
insist "Not true! Not true!" But our experience – as eyes glance off us,
through us, by us – makes menopause and aging indistinguishable.

A menopausal woman moves, quite suddenly and quite unexpectedly, from a category of "secondary person" (status based on
sex) to a category of "nonperson" (status based on age). This may
sound extreme, but let me explain. As a woman, one becomes
accustomed to throwaway lines that denigrate women: "She thinks
like a man," "Just like a woman!", and so on. Some of us have
learned to tune in to these kinds of remarks (many made quite
unconsciously) and to refute them. Those of us trained to examine

and analyze social values may feel some satisfaction in alerting others to these entrenched and sexist attitudes and, in so doing, limping toward the goal of equality between the sexes.

Then we run into ageism. It is difficult to combat social attitudes if you are neither heard nor seen. It is ageist when a sales clerk insists on serving everyone between the ages of twenty and forty before she condescends to help the sixty-year-old woman who got there first. It is ageist when doctors spend time explaining options to younger patients but then *tell* older patients what they must do. An aging person finds it more difficult to deal with ageism than sexism – he or she must first attract attention in order to point it out! It is not aging that is difficult. Much of the pain comes from banging against solid, unseen, and unexpected ageist attitudes in this society.

Men appear to age at a fairly steady rate. The changes in hair color and texture, the alterations in girth and visual acuity, the gradual decrease in energy level are incremental and barely noticeable. There are not many men who look thirty-five when they're close to fifty, and those who do will go to some pains to look their real age. The appearance of youth for a man is a disadvantage in a society dominated by middle-aged men.

Both the process and the prospect of aging are different for a woman. There are a great many women in their late forties who can easily pass for thirty-five. Because this knack of "not looking your age" is so admired, many women strive to look thirty-five for as long as possible. Some women just don't change much – a few laugh lines, a bit of gray at the temples – in the years from thirty-five to fifty. This resistance to the effects of aging, whether contrived or natural, sets the stage for what the French call *un coup de vieux* – aging overnight. Many women in their early fifties are plunged into despair because time suddenly catches up with them. At fifty-one or fifty-three, they finally look their age and, because they have looked thirty-five for so long, they appear to have aged fifteen years in five.

We live in a society that values women as decorative, sexual, and utilitarian. The first two are reserved for youth. Many of us find the third small comfort, although it helps us to be more understanding of the legions of middle-aged women who become involved in committee work for religious institutions or hospitals. The need to feel "useful" becomes urgent when one is devalued in other ways. If the paid and volunteer work of all women between fifty and sixty were withdrawn for twenty-four hours, just imagine what would happen!

The Need to Maintain Appearances

I feel that a valid role model for the middle-aged group is lacking. How can you call Joan Collins a role model, when the principal reason she is lauded is because she is *not* typical? I am one of those women who is fortunate enough to look younger than her age. I find myself frequently telling people how old I am so that I can see the surprise register on their faces and get the inevitable reassuring compliments about how I cannot possibly be that old. And all this because it feels *good* to get the reassurance that I don't look like what I am.

   I cannot feel good about myself when I am asking others to help me deny that I am what I inescapably am. I feel trapped by my looks. Trapped. When all I want to do is give up and be me (whoever that is).

Many middle-aged women have no clear idea of what it means to look one's age. Clothes, makeup, hairstyles are all modeled for us on much younger women. By showing us that this is the way we are *supposed* to look, we are told, over and over, that age is an enemy to be conquered. This is to strengthen us for the battle, but it also serves to emphasize the horror of aging – not only to women, but to everyone else. It is implied that any middle-aged woman could look like this model or that actress if only she *cared* enough. The truth is that the role models shown to us – aging actresses or winners of cosmetic manufacturers' contests – are individuals who, by dint of exercise, or cosmetic surgery, or genetics (or all three) do not look their age.

Exercise is beneficial. Each of us needs to have at least three hours of foot-pounding, arm-swinging exercise each week. This will enable our bones to remain strong. But it will not necessarily give us back the waistlines (and bustlines) of our youth. A dogged regimen of aerobics implies rewards, and Jane Fonda's videotapes and walking tapes implicitly promise a Jane Fonda shape. But Jane Fonda is built like Henry Fonda, and my father (and probably yours) wasn't built at all like Henry Fonda! We must approach exercise in light of its real benefits and not in search of an impossible dream.

When I was taking my first course in word processing, I suddenly discovered that the little flashing light (the cursor) would not move. I had been typing away quite merrily, when suddenly I couldn't get any more letters to jump onto the screen. I hit keys at random (there are many extra keys on the computer keyboard), and when nothing happened, I appealed to the teacher. She glanced quickly at the screen and said, "But you have a closed field." She then explained that since I hadn't given prior instructions to the computer, it wouldn't accept any additional information. It was not in the right "mode."

I've always thought that this was a perfect analogy to my situation at the time. I was learning to use a computer with a view to perhaps launching a newsletter about menopause and midlife. I was feeling very discouraged about myself – both in terms of appearance and frame of mind. My mother was urging me to tint my hair and I seemed to be moving into a larger dress size every few months. I had a clear idea of what kind of fortyish woman I'd been and of the feisty old lady I intended to be, but I had absolutely no idea of what kind of person I'd be for the next fifteen years. I was so aware of my years that I lapsed into self-disparagement, referring to myself as "a tired old woman" or "your old mother." (I winced when I heard myself, but I couldn't seem to stop it.) My field was "closed" – I couldn't find a realistic image of what I could be or what I wanted to be. I was suddenly confronting middle age and I didn't like it.

From the letters I receive, I know that my own escalation from size eight to size twelve is not unusual. I agonized about too-tight clothes for months, telling myself that the weight gain was because I had quit smoking; it had nothing to do with menopause. (This was, after all, what most of the books said.) I think now that stopping smoking was responsible for my weight gain, but the onset of menopause ensured that the weight stayed on. It took three years before I would look at myself, undressed, in a full-length mirror. Three years before I could begin to accept that the fat lady in the mirror was me.

Bodily changes

There is always a time lag when there is a physical change: the self-image (which is a purely mental construct) and the real image (what others see) may not jibe, and it takes time for these two images to match. This is true for those who lose a limb, those who lose weight, and those who gain it. It takes time to get used to the new shape, and the adaptation period may not be particularly pleasant. Don't try to jam yourself into too-tight clothes; this just accentuates the weight gain. Pack away the clothes that don't fit (they may fit one day!) and start acquiring larger sizes. It helps if you have some kind of idea of what you look like, so ask a trusted friend to point out women who resemble you in terms of height and overall shape. Chances are you will be pleasantly surprised to find you are not as gargantuan as you had imagined!

> The problem I encountered with menopause was not so much the weight gain as the inability to shed those extra pounds. I weighed between 120 and 125 for most of my life, and then, just as my periods started getting infrequent, I was up to 135! And it would *not* come off. I tried all the diets, and I have finally accepted that this extra poundage is inevitable. I've gradually acquired a new wardrobe, have joined a fitness class, and am truly feeling good about myself. I even think that the slight padding on my face makes me look better (but I don't know if everyone else agrees).

Remember that the extra pounds are providing extra estrogen, that the precursor for estrone, the most important estrogen post-menopausally, is converted *in your fatty tissue*, and that this process will not only protect you from hot flashes, but will do so more effectively with time. Remind yourself that underweight women are more likely to suffer from osteoporosis. Better to gain weight at menopause than to suddenly lose weight.

How you move inside your body is often more of a giveaway than shape. If you're discouraged by your new size, concentrate on keeping your body firm and flexible. If you're already involved in doing regular exercise (as outlined in chapter 8), you will be able to gracefully accommodate the extra weight. If you walk with a spring in your step, consciously adopting an air of confidence, others will react to you more positively. When I gained weight, I was frequently told how *well* I looked. I mourn my "lost" figure, but the added pounds have taken away dark circles from under my eyes and added a certain roundness of cheek!

The skin

If adolescence produces acne, then middle age produces dry skin. Most of us can now indulge in bath oils, lotions, and moisturizers without having to lock them away from the reach of experimenting daughters. There are numerous products on the market: upscale products that feature models with flawless (and poreless) skin; products aimed at "the wrinklies" and bins of products "on special" at the discount drugstore. The latter are probably as effective as any. Dermatologists recommend products containing petrolatum (Vaseline lotion, Nivea cream) or lanolin, and tell us to apply them while the skin is still damp. Rubbing Vaseline into the skin on your legs as you sit in a hot bath is as effective as using a high-priced body lotion. Buy soaps that have a minimal amount of perfume and detergent – clear soaps or Dove. Indulge yourself.

The skin changes in other ways. Many of us notice small red dots (cherry angiomas) appearing on the rib cage or stomach, or red threadlike marks (spider angiomas). Other marks appear – small reddish or purplish marks or the suddenly observed tracery of small blood vessels under the skin. (When we see broken veins on the legs – our own or anyone else's – we often think of them as varicose veins. This is often wrong; many of these are broken veins that can be removed quite easily. Look for an expert, often a medical doctor, in sclerotherapy. The Yellow Pages may have a listing.)

One of the most hated skin changes is the appearance of liver spots (senile lentigos), which have nothing to do with the liver at all but which show up on the back of the hands, on the arms or on the face – and which darken after exposure to the sun. Some women also notice patches of scaly, dark skin appearing on the chest or back. These "moles" feel oily and thick to the touch and are just one kind of mole that may appear. Others are flat, dark "beauty spots" or pale "skin tags" – light-colored moles that hang away from the skin, usually at places that are constantly rubbed by bra straps, or waistbands. All of these are normal. Tretinoin cream (Retin-A) is effective in fading liver spots: rub the cream onto the backs of the hands every night. The spots may take a few weeks to fade. Other types of undesirable spots can be removed by a dermatologist.

> All my life I've looked on gray hair and liver spots as signs
> of old age. These two superficial (when you think about it)
> changes in appearance signified the "end of youth" for me.
> I was really upset when I noticed liver spots developing on
> the backs of my hands. I'd handled the gray hair by regular
> sessions with the wash-in hair coloring, but liver spots! The
> only consolation I have is that after a summer of carefree
> sunning, a couple of my friends started moaning about their
> liver spots. Misery does love company.

As we age, our skin becomes more vulnerable to the ravages of the sun. Sunscreen is recommended for all ages, but it is imperative for both youngsters and oldsters, and it's wise to get in the habit of smoothing it on now. The skin changes to worry about are the various forms of skin cancer. Basal skin cancer starts with a pink, hairless, waxy-looking growth, usually on the head or neck, and changes over time to a cluster of shiny white pimples, then to a deep, crusted sore. Squamous cell cancer starts as a small, hard, red pimple and then becomes a crusted sore that refuses to heal – a sore with an irregular edge to it. Malignant melanoma (the cancer linked to imprudent and excessive exposure to the sun) starts as a slightly raised or bumpy, dark brown, black, or blue area of skin with irregular edges, usually more than 6 mm (1/4 in.) across, that changes in color, shape, or size and that may feel itchy or sore. These kinds of skin changes warrant an appointment with the doctor.

One of the most effective ways of encouraging healthy skin is to do more exercise. Many of us have found that the wintertime nuisance of dry, flaking skin on legs and arms can be noticeably modified by regular workouts. If you can afford it, regular body massage is both comforting and nourishing to the skin. It's remarkable how many gobs of lotion can be absorbed during a soothing massage.

The face

Wrinkling is caused not by the outer layer of skin (the epidermis), but by changes in the connective tissue of the dermis. With age, more and more of these connective fibers are produced, and as you smile, frown, or grimace, the outer layer of skin creases to fit against the excess mass underneath. As you age, these creases get worn into the skin: the elasticity of youth is no longer there.

Premature wrinkles are caused by smoking (which produces wrinkles fanning out from the lips or corners of the eyes) and, most of all, by sunbathing (which dries the outer layer of skin prematurely). Cosmetic advertising would have us believe that the wrinkling process can be arrested, but it can't. Most cosmetics that claim to "prevent new wrinkles" contain a sunscreen, which is necessary in the sun but which may come too late to prevent wrinkles that are already there. There are tretinoin creams (Renova, Retin-A, Vesanoid, etc.) which, used over a period of months, smooths out fine wrinkles and blurs darker patches from too much sun. It is available by prescription only.

Almost all soaps dry the skin because they remove skin lipids (fats) and the skin's own moisturizing substances. There are all sorts of skin cleansers on the market, but if you need soap to feel clean, dermatologists recommend a mild soap, followed by a moisturizer. Many suggest that the moisturizer be used on damp skin. Collagen-based cosmetics promise to restore the skin's *own* collagen (the protein that forms skin and bone), but the collagen actually comes from cows and the molecules are too large to get past the skin's outermost layer. Collagen injections can temporarily plump up skin and smooth out wrinkles, but this is a different matter entirely. If there is no adverse reaction to collagen (some women are allergic to it), the benefits will last from six to twelve months. The injections must be done by an experienced dermatologist or cosmetic surgeon.

Estrogen is often discussed as a "cure" for wrinkling. Women who are small boned and very fair often develop the kind of transparent skin, particularly on the back of the hands, that shows every vein. This often signals a serious depletion of collagen, not only in the underlying layers of skin but also in bone. These are the kind of women most susceptible to osteoporosis and some forms of arthritis, and ET is often prescribed to halt the loss of collagen or bone mass. Halting loss of collagen from the dermis, the underlying layer of skin, does not affect the outermost layer, the epidermis, which will still wrinkle.

The hair

The appearance of gray hair is, in our society, a marker of age. We envy those who are prematurely gray (seeing it as unusual and special) and those who retain their natural hair color into old age. Most of us can expect to have 50 percent of the hair on our head go gray by the age of fifty. And at least 50 percent of fifty-year-old women will choose not to let this show, opting instead for at-home rinse-in "tints" or regular visits to the beauty salon for more permanent hair coloring.

There's no doubt that gray hair reinforces the image of middle age. When I chose to go gray, the strongest argument I got against doing so was from my mother, who did not want an obviously middle-aged daughter! I decided to let nature take its course, however, because my hair was a natural auburn, which is almost impossible to reproduce; because it would take time and regular salon visits to keep it up, because the new gray hairs seemed softer and silkier than the natural red-brown "steel wool"; and – most important of all – because I was afraid I wouldn't know when to *stop* dying my hair. Whenever I went out, I would look for women who colored their hair: I saw too many who *should* have had gray hair but who were sporting false and/or harsh colors they had chosen years before. Who, I wondered, would come up to me and say, "Excuse me, my dear, but your hair color is so obviously false that you had better let your natural color show"? Also, I have to admit, my husband went gray *first*!

All of this is to illustrate that the decision to go gray or not is highly individual. And the decision often has to be made before there are significant gray hairs. Somehow the natural color turns drab and lifeless just as the gray starts to creep in, and, like it or not, you find yourself browsing the wash-in, nonperoxide products at the drugstore, looking for something to recapture the shine of healthy hair. Women who eat nutritious foods and exercise regularly may be less affected by this premenopausal drabness, but this is when most of us start seriously considering whether to use rinses or dyes.

Because gray hair is often finer, not always, the gray tide may also bring an unwelcome thinning with most women noticing a reduction of about 30 percent in volume of hair. Tinting the hair coats the hair shaft and adds body if thinning is minor. Often there is a family tendency to thinning hair, and often this happens in families where hair tends to be fine in texture to start with. Some postmenopausal women are affected by "male pattern baldness" and find the hair thinning either at the temples or at the crown of the head. This is assumed to be due to the effects of adrenal hormones that are no longer being counteracted by ovarian hormones. Until recently, nothing much could be done about this. Minoxidil, originally developed to alleviate high blood pressure, is now available by prescription as Rogaine. It is expensive, it only works for 30 to 40 percent of those who try it, it must be rubbed on the scalp indefinitely to be effective, and it is too early to assess long-term effects. (If a woman suffers from patchy hair loss, this may be alopecia areata, a condition not linked to menopause.)

My hair, although fine, has never been a problem. As a matter of fact, it has always been very healthy and certainly plentiful. In the last six months, it has been falling out at an alarming rate. My husband seems to think I'm overreacting, but I figure I know my hair best, and this is really scaring me! It's not only that it's falling out – it's coming out in patches. In other words, I'm losing hair in places like around my temples. I'm beginning to wonder if this problem is related to menopause.

Beauticians suggest that hair color should not mimic natural color; in most cases, the color chosen should be lighter. Ash blond may be too drab; deep brunette is probably too harsh. You might take a tip from young people and their hair of many colors: experiment with some of the new brush-in colors that disappear after one shampoo. If you are trying a nonperoxide rinse, choose a shade close to your natural color but warmer, then gradually lighten the shade. Because one of these rinses lasts for a few weeks, the gradual change will probably not even be noticed. Keep your hair short – shoulder length at the longest – and use soft bangs or wisps of hair over the forehead and an uplift at the sides. Avoid backcombing, hair lacquer, or outdated "bouffant" styles. Hair mousse adds body without changing the color and can be combed into the hair each morning, if necessary. Another way of adding body is the body perm, which can be done at home, provided you use very large plastic rollers, larger than those supplied with the standard home permanent kit.

It's unsettling to have to deal with these kinds of changes. My hair, which had once been very wavy, became quite unmanageable for a few years, and I ended up having a series of curly perms because I was so awkward with a hair dryer and curling iron. Now that it is gray, the wave has returned, and I have gone back to finger-combing it after a shampoo. In fact, in humid weather, my hair is wavier than it's been since I was a teenager. The analogy between menopause and adolescence holds, even for hair!

In addition to scalp hair, we must also deal with body hair and facial hair. Most of us notice a thinning of body hair – more and more infrequent shaving of the underarms, less need to shave the legs. On the other hand, the tweezers are needed more and more for stray chin hairs, and for women who tend to be dark and hairy (hirsute) anyway, there may be the ominous shadow of a mustache. Of course, this whole idea of being hairless is a *learned* standard and quite silly when you think about it. There is no doubt that this society likes its women hairless to emphasize the childlike aspects of womanhood, whereas some societies find hairy women very sexy. Interesting how one can see this so plainly, yet feel compelled to banish all evidence of hair on the face, legs, and armpits!

Facial hairs seem to get worse during the menopause, then to ease up afterward. I noticed that the whiskers appeared on a cyclical basis, even after I stopped menstruating: for one week of the month, I would feel them, get rid of them, and worry that my face would one day be covered in stubble. Now I find the whiskers appear only rarely. So don't panic if you are tweezing whiskers regularly. This may resolve itself in time.

Be aware, however, that certain drugs – some hypertensive medications, diuretics, antidepressants, and tranquilizers – encourage the growth of facial hair. Don't blame it all on menopause. Estrogen may diminish hair growth but should not be considered (or prescribed) for this reason alone. Spironolactone (Aldactone, Sincomen, etc.), an antiandrogen and diuretic, has occasionally been prescribed in low doses to reduce growth of heavy facial hair, although it takes some time for the effects to be seen. Medication should be a last resort; spironolactone may also inhibit sex drive and cause nausea, cramping, diarrhea, drowsiness, headaches, and other unpleasant side effects. There is also some concern about possible long-term effects.

If facial hair is fair, tweezing may be the simplest solution; you will need a good magnifying mirror in a place with a strong light. If the hair is fine but dark, you may want to invest in facial bleach, which is readily available at a drugstore; the instructions are easy to follow. If the hair is dark and sturdy, you may want to try a new depilatory for facial hair, or remove it (or have it removed) with wax; there are cold-wax and hot-wax methods. There are also special devices available that pull out the offending hairs and that claim to lead to permanent hairlessness. Check at your local drugstore. Another permanent solution is electrolysis, which kills individual follicles using an electric current. It has to be done by a skilled operator and will require a number of sessions.

Many malls have boutiques that sell cosmetics and also offer free makeup sessions. I tried this once and received a lot of useful tips. Because these malls are bathed in artificial light, the amount of makeup applied is often too garish for daylight hours, but it may give you confidence in making up for swank evening events where you want to look your best and the lighting will tolerate a heavier hand. I bought some of the small brushes in return for my "free makeup session" – a fair trade, I thought. For women committed to the natural look, the use of makeup just takes up time and money. But for those of us who like a touch of artifice, self-enhancement becomes a challenge.

The smile

More and more of us are looking to dentists to improve our appearance. Some of this is involuntary as we all get "longer in the tooth" – literally as well as figuratively – and the periodontists get to work on our defective gums. Some dental work is optional and cosmetic. It is no longer unusual to see women of forty or fifty wearing braces on their teeth, and orthodontists are attracting more middle-aged customers by offering sapphire braces, which are almost invisible. Even more numerous are those women who have their teeth bonded to get rid of unsightly spots, the marks of old fillings, or to minimize small chips or gaps. Dentists are also offering teeth-whitening programs. They are expensive – $600 or more – and, sad to say, work better on younger teeth.

Cosmetic surgery

I resent those who look down their noses at the idea of cosmetic surgery. It's no more artificial to extend the youthful appearance of the face with a facelift than it is to extend the elasticity of the vagina with an estrogen cream. I suspect a moral judgment at work here: vanity (self) is bad, sexual accessibility (other) is good. A love of beauty is by no means the worst part of us. I don't subscribe to the notion that lines are necessarily an indication of character. Lines are an indication of lines.

Not all women are interested in having cosmetic surgery; not all of us are candidates, because a number of medical conditions dictate against it (hypertension, heart disease, diabetes), and not all of us can afford it. When we think of cosmetic surgery, facelifts immediately come to mind. But more and more women are turning to cosmetic surgery for a body lift.

Body contouring, as it's euphemistically known, is not a substitute for dieting or exercise. In fact, it is not recommended for those whose weight tends to fluctuate. The ideal candidate for this operation has localized areas of excessive fat, an otherwise normal and fairly stable body weight, and good skin elasticity. Where skin has lost this elasticity (a natural effect of aging), a complementary operation to remove excess skin (an abdominoplasty or tummy tuck) may be performed – either at the same time or some weeks later.

Fat suction (also known as liposuction, suction curettage, lipectomy, or lipolysis) is done under either local or general anesthetic, depending on the extent and duration of surgery. Fat suction of the abdomen requires three incisions: one at each end of the pubic crease and another at the navel. For pads of fat under the breasts or on the sides of the waist, additional incisions may be required. A long-handled looped instrument is inserted into each incision and moved around to break up the cells, then a miniature wand (similar to the extension on a vacuum cleaner but much smaller, of course) is inserted and moved about under the top layer of skin to suck out the fat.

After the fat has been vacuumed off, drains may be inserted and incisions closed with a suture. Or the incisions may be left open for additional drainage after the drains are removed (twenty-four to forty-eight hours post-surgery). The patient is permitted to walk the evening after surgery and to shower forty-eight hours after the operation. The hospital or clinic stay will be from two to five days, with pressure dressings required for three weeks and, for older patients, an abdominal girdle for a week or two after that. Patients can usually resume normal activity in a week to ten days, and heavy exercise in three to four weeks. A change is noticeable within three weeks of the operation, but because damaged cells will continue to be sloughed off for some time, it may take a month or two for the full benefits to show.

Severe bruising follows from the operation, but the extent and duration of the bruises will depend on age, coloring, and other factors. There is often a "rippling" effect on the skin – in other words, the skin does not necessarily go back to the smooth contours of youth. If the rippling is still unacceptable a month or two after the operation, a second procedure to smooth out excess skin may be required. Potential side effects are necrosis (death of clumps of cells), which may require additional surgery, and unexpected and disfiguring scars.

Fat suction may seem like an easy solution to abdominal padding, but there are disadvantages at menopause. The ethical plastic surgeon wants to operate on a person whose body weight is relatively stable and who will, therefore, derive a long-term benefit. For many menopausal women, the change in shape (whether or not it involves a weight change) is only part of the picture. Often there are fluctuations in energy levels or temporary feelings of anxiety, panic, or even depression. In such a state of flux, the trauma of anesthesia combined with the shock of surgery may merely *add* to the physiological strain, putting *more* stress on a body already under siege. A well-known New York cosmetic surgeon has commented that such operations "buy time" for the woman not prepared to deal with the reality of aging. My own feeling is that it is better to confront aging and then, when you're feeling good about yourself, to reward yourself with a smoother forehead or a flatter tummy.

About 10 percent of cosmetic surgeries entail some unexpected and negative outcome. Surgeons are responsible for the conduct of the surgical procedure, but there is no guarantee of satisfactory results. For this reason, any woman seeking surgical treatment should be very wary. Make sure you are dealing with a reputable surgeon. See the Resources section for medical associations that can provide names of qualified surgeons in your area of the country.

No matter what kind of operation you choose, you should get a referral or recommendation from a family physician or from former patients who have had the same operation. Doctors who are affiliated with a hospital must conform to certain hospital standards in order to use those facilities. If the doctor practices in a private clinic, you may want to check to see if he or she *did*, at one time, have hospital privileges. If the doctor has a university appointment or is with a teaching hospital, this is usually considered a plus.

When you see the doctor, ask how many similar procedures he or she has performed and when. If the doctor is evasive – "Don't you worry about that. I know my business" – excuse yourself. Any surgeon should be willing to answer this question frankly and honestly. If you don't know anyone who has undergone the same procedure, ask to see photographic results of other operations. If former patients are willing to be contacted, ask to get in touch with them. The more information you have, the better.

Before you start your investigations you should be aware that because the surgery is for cosmetic purposes, it will not be covered by medicare and thus can be very expensive. The exception is breast reduction, which may be covered.

Last spring I had a facelift. This was not common knowledge, but my close friends knew about it, and a couple of them came down hard on me for deciding to go ahead with it. It's funny, because although I had severe misgivings about "postponing" the aging process, I feel I am benefiting from the operation.

As women, we are continually reminded of the importance of our looks. It seems odd, then, that after years of emphasis on makeup and clothes, we're chided for trying to improve ourselves when we get to fifty or fifty-five. Granted it's a drastic and costly step, but I found it made a difference in my attitude to myself and, I think, in the attitude of my students toward me. I guess I look more "with it" now so they seem to pay more attention to what I have to say. Or maybe I'm just imagining it!

The ultimate solution to the specter of aging is, of course, the facelift. This procedure (rhytidectomy) requires a hospital or clinic stay of from one to three days, another week of isolation, and three more weeks before the swelling disappears completely. The effects last for five to eight years. An incision is made in the scalp behind the hairline at the temple, descending to the front of the ear and back up behind the ear. If neck tissue is to be removed, the incision will extend downward from behind the ear and into the neck. Possible complications are hematomas (swellings containing blood), which occur in from 10 to 15 percent of cases and which must be drained. In addition, it is impossible to predict changes in skin pigmentation or the kind of scarring that may result. In rare cases, injury may be caused to a facial nerve.

Chemical face peeling is a procedure that burns off the top layer of skin and that is often used to remove fine wrinkles around the mouth and eyes. It takes from four to twelve weeks for the skin to appear normal, and you will have to stay out of the sun for a full year. Possible long-term effects are scarring or changes in skin coloring. Dermabrasion is often mentioned as an alternative to chemical face peeling, but it's more useful for acne scars than for wrinkles.

For pouches under the eyes or hooded eyelids, some women resort to the eyelift or blepharoplasty. The operation for the lower eyelid is more difficult and, if done improperly, may prevent the eye from closing properly. Eye surgery usually involves an overnight stay at a hospital or clinic and can be done under local anesthesia. The patient must keep a compress on the eyes for at least ten hours, often longer, and this is usually the part of the procedure most difficult to tolerate. It takes about ten days to recover and two months before the final effect is achieved.

For bags under the eyes that are primarily composed of fat, a technique uses an electrically heated needle to vaporize the fat. Done under local anesthetic, this procedure takes about thirty minutes and heals in about a week. Plastic surgeons can use this same procedure to remove pads of fat under the chin. A nonsurgical solution to hooded eyelids is a piece of medical adhesive that is specially designed to hold up the kind of eyelids that fold right down to, or past, the eyelashes. This product can be used daily.

Makeup and fashion

Whether or not you choose to spend money and time on cosmetic surgery, you still want to look your best. When you start to notice a loss of luster or color in your hair (whether tinted or not), you will also notice changes in skin color. If you continue to use the same makeup colors and techniques at forty-five as you used at thirty-five, you are probably doing yourself a disservice. The experts say that as you age you should conscientiously try to be more deft, more subtle with makeup, matching foundation carefully to skin color and abandoning rouge for a carefully dusted-on contouring powder.

Soft pencil can be used under the eye and along the upper lid, but it should be softened or smudged to avoid a hard line. Reddish brown or pinkish brown eye shadow is more natural than turquoise or blue. If you wear glasses, you can use more eye makeup because glasses soften the effect.

For cracked or chapped lips, use a lip balm, wipe to remove dead skin, then use a lip primer to prevent "bleeding" of lipstick into lip creases. These primers are expensive, but they last a long time. A lip pencil will also help to keep the lipstick inside the lines. Also, as small wrinkles appear around the mouth, any lip line that does not follow the natural lip line appears more and more false. Softer lipstick shades are more flattering to the midlife woman; they put less emphasis on the mouth, and more attention is drawn toward the wise and worldly eyes!

We are fortunate in that fashion options are so wide these days. Despite the announcements that "waists are nipped" or "skirts are shorter," we can pick and choose in a way not available to midlife women twenty or thirty years ago. Coping with bodily changes means more than buying the same old thing but in a larger size. A skirt hangs differently over a budding tummy and the waistband cuts during a temporary episode of "bloat." It seemed strange to feel my panty hose, panties, and skirts all clinging to different parts of my middle; my waist seemed to be everywhere and nowhere.

Not long ago, I read the remark of a fashion expert: "Middle-aged women will love the shorter skirts because the legs are the last to go." Despite the anger I felt at this woman's patronizing remark, I had to admit that there was a grain of truth. Few of us worry about gaining weight on our legs. There is a tendency for weight to accumulate around the waist, on the diaphragm, across the back – a different story from the heavy hips and thighs that are common problem areas at younger ages.

Midlife women need elasticized waistbands, pleats that are stitched down to the hip or that fall from a yoke, big tops that sit easily on the hips or skim down to the old "three-quarter" length. We need bright touches of color to cheer us up and to flatter our changing hair and skin color. How many of us tune into reruns of *The Golden Girls*, not for the story line, but to get ideas for suitable clothes?

✦

Women are motivated to seek adjustments to their appearance for a number of reasons. Some are touched by the "now-or-never" syndrome – the same syndrome that incites a midlife woman to leave a marriage or to start a business. These women will go in search of the straight teeth, the firm chin, the wide-open eyes that they have fantasized about for years. Other women find that their physical appearance just does not *fit* with their personalities; for them, worn wrappings do not fairly represent the up-to-date contents.

These may not be the women you think of in connection with cosmetic surgery, but they are as much a part of the picture as the common stereotype of the woman frightened of aging, the woman who blindly seeks help from a surgeon rather than confronting her own nightmares. We rarely notice the surgical enhancement of the stable woman; what we remark on are the aging women with the incongruously young faces. The tragedy of such women is that their movements and attitudes are so antiquated, so aging, that the facelifts are merely grotesque.

Because the aged are devalued in this society, most of us find any evidence of aging unwelcome. In one study of middle-agers, more than one-third voluntarily cited changes in physical appearance as a concern. There is no doubt that for many women menopause brings many changes; it's not easy to cope with a new shape and a new image. But if we're realistic about it, we will acknowledge that it is not being fifty that bothers us, but rather the prospect of being viewed as "old." If menopause is on the doorstep of old age, then we have to confront our fear of aging.

> I'm very conscious of getting older. I don't really want to be old. I'd like to put the clock back to about forty and stop there, because although I enjoyed the children when they were little, at forty I was enjoying my job. I was on top of the world. I was full of bounce ... I'm a bit afraid now that I'm over fifty. I can see sixty coming and I really feel that that is very old ...
>
> I can see retirement, and although my husband says we'll go around the world and all sorts of things, my fear is that by the time we're old enough to do these things, we won't be young enough to enjoy them. I'm afraid that I will deteriorate very quickly when I get older.
>
> I'm afraid that tiredness is going to stay with me and, in fact, increase. That really frightens me. I can't bear to think of not being well. I don't mind being old so long as I'm well.

The Need to Confront Our Own Aging

For many of us, growing old means not being needed. We all want a little niche where our presence will be noted, appreciated, and, in our absence, missed. Many women's lives are unbalanced from being needed too much for too long, then suddenly needed too little. One friend, who has been forced to move away from her grown children and back to the place where her husband wants to grow old, says it has put her "off balance." Not much wonder. It requires enormous resilience to cope with a social worth that can so quickly redefine one from "essential" to "nonessential."

Years ago, I was pushing our baby carriage toward the house. In the carriage was my new baby girl and her seventeen-month-old brother. On a little chair fitted over the carriage sat my eldest, not quite three. Rain was threatening and I was about to break into a trot, when a little old lady stopped me, peered into the carriage, and said sweetly, "Ah, my dear, these are the best years of your life!" I remember the rage I felt that anyone should label these the "best" years of my life – years of constant fatigue and incredible self-doubt. What a price to pay for being needed! (It made for a nice irony when, twenty-five years later, I was part of a National Film Board video entitled *The Best Time of My Life: Portraits of Women in Midlife*.) Is it possible to designate any years as the "best"?

There are different ways of being needed. We may fulfill basic needs (food, clothing, shelter, love) or we may fulfill secondary needs (advice, friendship, affection, touching). If we spend a large part of our lives dispensing love with hot meals and clean clothes, we sometimes confuse them. We fear that when we are no longer needed to cook, shop, and "do" for others, we will no longer be needed. But we are needed to love them, as we have always done. It is normal to feel a sense of loss when one role ends and another has yet to begin. The gap created may leave us "off balance," but not, I hope, too timid to reach out to others who need us – who need our advice, our friendship, our touch. We *can* make a place for ourselves at this age, as at any age. The gap closes.

Closely allied to the fear of not being needed is the fear of having no central objective or purpose to one's life. Menopause often coincides with other major events in a woman's life – the end of "active" mothering, the awarding of the twenty-five-year pin to the faithful employee, the sudden and saddening loss of a parent or spouse, the growing awareness that one may be destined to spend old age alone. Those of us who thought that we would feel great satisfaction when we surveyed our grown children find instead that their growing-up years have become a blur. These young adults, fine as they are, seem to have appeared out of nowhere. Now, married, separated, divorced, or widowed, we have to look for new means to achieve satisfaction, the sense of a job well done.

At the same time, there is often a sense of being very *tired*, too tired to undertake anything new or different. You may just want to be left alone. I believe that this fatigue has its reasons. The body is adapting to a new internal rhythm and you need time to rest and to think. Middle age allows time for the reactivation of old dreams, the challenges of new learning, the tentative acquisition of new skills. When your energy comes flowing back – as it will – you will have found a cause, an activity, a source of satisfaction that will give meaning to what you do for the next major stage in your life.

It is during this pause, the real gift of middle age, that we should take time to examine our fears of aging. Today, confronted with new facts about the patterns and prevalence of Alzheimer's disease, we find ourselves nervously joking about menopausal forgetfulness, dying brain cells, premature senility, but there is often a deadly serious edge to our humor. We fumble for names, lose objects that turn up in the most mysterious places, notice that every stranger we meet looks like someone else (are we really that old?), and remember arcane bits of information from childhood. Psychologists tell us that this is a different kind of memory, no better and no worse than the memory of youth. They also tell us that women (who are usually held responsible for remembering the trivia of everyday life) worry far more about loss of memory than do men, although the changes in memory are similar. Victims of Alzheimer's rarely worry about loss of memory, because one of the symptoms of the disease is the inability to realize that you have forgotten something.

Like the fear of forgetting, the fear of becoming dependent is often expressed in black humor – for instance, the T-shirts and bumper stickers sold in Florida: 'Avenge yourself. Live long enough to be a burden to your children.' No one wants to be dependent, and this is one of the greatest fears of aging. Most of us know old people so haunted by this fear that it can never be spoken. There are no discussions, no contingency plans.

If this fear dogs you, take this time to examine your economic future. The government listings in the telephone book can guide you to information about pension plans. If you have a pension plan at work, you should be getting regular statements of your pension status. You can discuss this with your bank manager and augment it, if possible, with RRSPs (Registered Retirement Savings Plans) or other forms of savings. If you are dependent on your husband's pension, make sure you know what the provisions are.

There are, of course, other forms of dependence aside from financial dependence. Many of us are frightened by the prospect of having to depend on others for routine help – shopping, driving, fixing things around the house. In our determination to take care of ourselves, we often forget the joy that comes from giving. There is a time to give and a time to allow others to give to us. In the meantime, we can do our best to assure our independence by assiduous attention to healthy living. By taking good care of ourselves now, we may ease the minds of our children and lighten the burden of those who will have to take care of us in our old age.

Middle age gives us a marvelous opportunity to prepare for being old. We have time to dream about, and to plan for, the future. Even if we are feeling under strain right now, we can anticipate years of good health and renewed energy that will enable us to get involved in new projects and new causes. We have the mental acuity, flexibility, and experience to deal with shifting relationships and with generations both older and younger. We have the freedom to adopt new eating patterns or new activities that may very well keep us healthy for years to come.

✦

I am often asked about the *good* things about menopause. It isn't hard to find them. First is the sense of freedom. We are free to experiment with new kinds of foods, new kinds of activities. We are free from having to stock sanitary pads or tampons or to schedule events around the ups-and-downs of the menstrual cycle. We are free to strike up a conversation with a stranger in a bus or on a street corner without being thought of as forward or seductive. We are free from the compulsion to work toward thinner thighs, or a twenty-four-inch waistline, or the perfect fingernails that we once longed for, and we are free to realize that those were pretty silly ambitions anyway! We are free to adopt our own standards of dress and decorum, guided more by good sense and comfort than by "What will people think?"

Then there is the sense of getting another chance. Because menopause often brings us up short, psychologically and physiologically, it gives us a rare opportunity to evaluate where we are coming from and where we want to go. Because of this enforced disruption, many of us have found that we were continuing to do things that we didn't really enjoy. They were part of the routine and we hadn't stopped to think about them. Every day, middle-aged women are giving up cooking to take up woodworking; are boycotting movies in order to save for trips to faraway places; are signing up for piano lessons, or computer science or philosophy courses. Women are making changes that are not perhaps significant in themselves, but that allow for the expression of very personal interests – interests that sometimes have been lurking beneath the surface for years.

Finally, menopause gives women an opportunity to make friends. Because so little is known about the causes and effects of menopause, the only real understanding of it comes from other women. Menopause provides the perfect excuse to reach out to other women – to revive old friendships and to forge new ones. We know that the nourishment that comes from friendship is a vital ingredient for a happy old age. We know that women are much more likely to survive into old age than are men. Thanks to menopause, we can enrich our lives now and carry these riches with us into an active and satisfying future.

SELECTED

REFERENCES AND

RESOURCES

Chapter 1

Backstrom, C.T., H. Boyle, and D.T. Baird. "Persistence of symptoms of premenstrual tension in hysterectomized women." *British Journal of Obstetrics and Gynecology*, 88:530–536, May 1981.

Cattanach, J. "Oestrogen deficiency after tubal ligation." *Lancet*, 1:847–849, April 1985.

Coulson, C.J. "Premenstrual syndrome: Are gonadotropins the cause of the condition?" *Medical Hypothesis*, 19:243–255, 1986.

Cramer, D.W., H. Xu, and B.L. Harlow "Family history as a predictor of early menopause." *Fertility & Sterility*, 64:740–745, 1995.

Cramer, D.W., H. Xu, and B.L. Harlow. "Does 'incessant' ovulation increase risk for early menopause?" *American Journal of Obstetrics & Gynecology*, 172:568–573, 1995.

Dalton, K. *The Premenstrual Syndrome and Progesterone Therapy.* 2nd ed. Chicago: Year Book Medical Publishers, 1984.

McKinlay, S., M. Jeffreys, and B. Thompson. "An investigation of the age at menopause." *Journal of Biosocial Science*, 4:161–173, 1972.

Riedel, H.H., E. Lehmann-Willenbrock, and K. Semm. "Ovarian failure after hysterectomy." *Journal of Reproductive Medicine*, 31:597–600, 1986.

Siddle, N., P. Sarrel, and M. Whitehead. "The effect of hysterectomy on the age at ovarian failure: Identification of a subgroup of women with premature loss of ovarian function and literature review." *Fertility and Sterility*, 47(1), January 1987.

Chapter 2

Ballinger, S.E. "A comparison of life stresses and symptomatology of menopause clinic patients and non-patients," Paper presented at the 4th International Congress on the Menopause, Buena Vista, Florida, 1984.

Cobb, J.O. "Fibromyalgia: The sore-all-over syndrome." *A Friend Indeed*, 7(9), February 1991.

Dudley, R., and W. Rowland. *How to Find Relief from Migraine.* Toronto: Collins, 1982.

Feldman, B.M., A.M. Voda, and E. Gronseth. "The prevalence of hot flash and associated variables among perimenopausal women." *Research in Nursing and Health,* 8:261–268, 1985.

Gillespie, L. *You Don't Have to Live with Cystitis.* New York: Avon Books, 1996.

Ginsburg, J., and P. Hardiman. "The menopausal hot flush: facts and fancies." *The Modern Management of the Menopause,* Berg & Hammar, eds. London: Parthenon Publishing, 1994.

Grushka, M., B.J. Sessle, and R. Miller. "Pain and personality profiles in burning mouth syndrome." *Journal of Pain,* 28(2):155–167, February 1987.

"Hair, Beautiful Hair." University of Toronto Faculty of Medicine *Health News,* 6(4):1–5, August 1988.

Kronenberg, F. "Hot flashes." *Treatment of the Postmenopausal Woman,* Lobo, ed. New York: Raven Press, 1994.

Kronenberg, F., L.J. Cote, and D.M. Linkie. "Menopausal hot flashes: Thermoregulatory, cardiovascular and circulating catecholamine and LH changes." *Maturitas,* 6(1):31–43, 1984.

Migraine Foundation, 365 Bloor St. E., Suite 1912, Toronto, Ontario M4W 3L4. Telephone (800) 663-3557 or (416) 920-4916.

Notelovitz, M., and M. Ware. *Stand Tall: The Informed Woman's Guide to Preventing Osteoporosis.* Florida: Triad Publishing, 1982.

Price, V.H. "Women and hair loss: Alopecia areata." *National Women's Health Report,* 3(5), May 1985.

Sacks, O. *Migraine: Evolution of a common disorder.* London: Faber and Faber, 1970.

Voda, A.M. "Menopausal hot flash." In *Changing Perspectives on Menopause.* Voda et al., eds. Austin, TX: University of Texas Press, 1982.

Voda, A.M., B.M. Feldman, and E. Gronseth. "Description of the hot flash: Sensations, meaning and change in frequency across time." Paper presented at the 4th International Congress on the Menopause, Buena Vista, Florida, 1984.

Waxman J., S.McS. Zatzkis. "Fibromyalgia and menopause." *Postgraduate Medicine* 80 (4), Sept. 15, 1986.

Woods, N.F. "Menopausal distress: A model for epidemiological investigation." In *Changing Perspectives on Menopause,* Voda et al., eds. Austin, TX: University of Texas Press, 1982.

Chapter 3

Albers, M.M. "Osteoporosis: A health issue for women." *Health Care for Women International,* 11:11–19, 1990.

Brown J.S., G. Sawaya et al. "Hysterectomy and urinary incontinence: A systematic review." *Lancet* 356:535–539, 2000.

Burgio, Kathryn L., K. Lynette Pearce, and Angelo J. Lucco. *Staying Dry: A Practical Guide to Bladder Control.* Baltimore, MD: The Johns Hopkins University Press, 1990.

Ditkoff, E.C., W.G. Crary, M. Cristo et al. "Estrogen improves psychological function in asymptomatic postmenopausal women." *Obstetrics & Gynecology* 78(6): 991–995, 1991.

Fantl, J.A., J.F. Wyman, R.L. Anderson et al. "Postmenopausal urinary incontinence: Comparison between nonestrogen-supplemented and estrogen-supplemented women." *Obstetrics and Gynecology*, 71(6), June 1988.

Gannon, L. "The potential role of exercise in the alleviation of menstrual disorders and menopause symptoms: A theoretical syntheses of recent research." *Women and Health*, 14(2):105–127, 1988.

Gillespie, L. *You Don't Have to Live with Cystitis.* New York: Avon Books, 1996.

Greendale, G.A., B.A. Reboussin, P. Hogan et al. "Symptom relief and side effects of postmenopausal hormones: results from the Postmenopausal Estrogen/Progestin Interventions (PEPI) Trial." *Obstetrics & Gynecology* 92 (6): 982–988, 1988.

Lieberman S. "A review of the effectiveness of *cimicifuga racemosa* (black cohosh) for the symptoms of menopause." *Journal of Women's Health* 7(5):525–529, 1998.

ICA *Update*, quarterly newsletter available from the Interstitial Cystitis Association, P.O. Box 1553, Madison Square Station, New York, NY 10159.

The Informer, quarterly newsletter on incontinence available from the Simon Foundation, P.O. Box 264, Station E, Toronto, Ontario M6H 4E2. Telephone (800) 265-9575.

NAFC (National Association for Continence) Report, quarterly newsletter available from HIP, Inc., Box 544, Union, SC 29379 (Resource guide and other publications also available.)

Polo-Kantola, P., R. Portin, O. Polo et al. "The effect of short-term estrogen replacement therapy on cognition: a randomized, double-blind, cross-over trial in postmenopausal women." *Obstetrics & Gynecology* 91 (3):459–466, 1998.

Ross, L.A., E.M. Alder, E.H. Cawood et al. "Psychological effects of hormone replacement therapy: a comparison of tibolone and a sequential estrogen therapy." *Journal of Psychosomatic Obstetrics & Gynecology* 20(2): 88–96, 1999.

Sherwin, B.B. "Estrogen and/or androgen replacement therapy and cognitive functioning in surgical menopausal women." *Psychoneuroendocrinology*, 13:345–357, 1988.

Sleep/Wake Disorders Canada, P.O. Box 223, Station S, Toronto, Ontario M5M 4L7. Telephone: (800) 387-9253 or (416) 398-1627.

Smith, W. *Overcoming Cystitis: A Practical Self-Help Guide for Women.* New York: Bantam Books, 1986.

South, Valerie. *Migraine.* Toronto: Key Porter, 1994.

"Test points out high-risk postmenopausal women" and "Calcium supplements: Role reassessed." In meeting highlights from the International Symposium on Osteoporosis, Aalborg, Denmark: *Geriatrics, 43*(5);90, May 1988.

Wolf, O.T., B.M. Kudielka, D.H. Hellhammer et al. "Two weeks of transdermal estradiol treatment in postmenopausal elderly women and its effect on memory and mood: Verbal memory changes are associated with the treatment induced estradiol levels." *Psychoneuroendocrinology* 24(7):727–741, 1991.

Chapter 4

Ballinger, S.E. "A comparison of life stresses and symptomatology of menopause clinic patients and nonpatients." Paper presented at the 4th International Congress on the Menopause, Buena Vista, Florida, 1984.

Barbach, L., and L. Levine. *Shared Intimacies: Women's Sexual Experiences.* New York: Wellness Institute, 2000.

Belenky, M.F., B.M. Clinchy, N.R. Goldberger, and J.M. Tarule. *Women's Ways of Knowing: The Development of Self, Voice, and Mind.* New York: Basic Books, 1997.

Campbell, B.C. and J.R. Udry. "Implications of hormonal influences on sexual behavior for demographic models of reproduction." *Annals of the New York Academy of Science,* 1994; 709:117–127.

Channon, L.S., and S.E. Ballinger. "Some aspects of sexuality and vaginal symptoms during menopause and their relation to anxiety and depression." *British Journal of Medical Psychology,* 59:173–180, 1986.

Chesler, P. *Women and Madness.* New York: Doubleday, 1972.

Cole, Ellen. "Sex at menopause: Each in her own way." In *Women and Sex Therapy: Closing the Circle of Sexual Knowledge,* Cole and Rothblum, eds. Binghamton, NY: Haworth Press, 1996.

Cole, Ellen, and Esther Rothblum. "Lesbian sex at menopause: As good or better than ever." In *Lesbians at Midlife: The Creative Transition,* Sang, Warshow, and Smith, eds. San Francisco: Spinsters Book Company, 1991.

Donovan, M.E., and L.T. Sanford. *Women and Self-Esteem.* New York: Doubleday, 1984.

Johnson, K. "Women and depression." *Medical Self Care,* 28:15, Spring 1985.

Kampen, D.L., and B.B. Sherwin. "Estrogen use and verbal memory in healthy postmenopausal women." *Obstetrics & Gynecology,* 83:979–983, 1994.

Kitzinger, S. *Women's Experience of Sex.* New York: Viking Press, 1985.

Lax, R. "The expectable depressive climacteric reaction." *Bulletin of the Menninger Clinic,* 46,(2):151–167, 1982.

Lerner, H.G. *The Dance of Anger.* New York: Harper Collins, 1997; and *The Dance of Intimacy.* New York: Harper Collins, 1990.

Lewisohn, P.M., et al. "Age at first onset for nonbipolar depression." *Journal of Abnormal Psychology,* 95(4):378–383, 1986.

Mansfield, P.K., A.M. Voda, and P.B. Koch. "Midlife sexual response changes: Effects of menopausal transition and context." Unpublished paper.

Masters, W., V. Johnson, and R. Kolodny. *Human Sexuality,* 2nd ed. Boston: Little Brown, 1985.

Matthews, K.A., R.R. Wing, L.H. Kuller et al. "Influences of natural menopause on psychological characteristics and symptoms of middle-aged healthy women." *Journal of Consulting and Clinical Psychology,* 58(3):345–351, 1990.

McCann, L., and D.S. Holmes. "Influence of aerobic exercise on depression." *Journal of Personal and Social Psychology,* 46:1142–1147, 1984.

McCoy, N.L., and J.M. Davidson. "A longitudinal study of the effects of menopause on sexuality." *Maturitas,* 17:203–210, 1985.

McKinlay, J.B., and N. Bifano. "Does the menopause cause depression in normally aging women?" Paper presented to the Society for Epidemiological Research, Durham, NC, 1985.

Philipp, M., R. Kohnen, K-O. Heller. "Hypericum extract [St. John's wort] vs. imipramine or placebo in patients with moderate depression; randomized multi-centre study of treatment for eight weeks." *British Medical Journal* 319:1534–1539, 1999.

Scarf, M. *Unfinished Business: Pressure Points in the Lives of Women.* New York: Ballantine, 1989.

Sherwin, B.B. "Changes in sexual behaviour as a function of plasma sex steroid levels in postmenopausal women." *Maturitas,* 7:225(1985).

Sherwin, B.B., M.M. Gelfand, and W. Brender. "Androgen enhances sexual motivation in females: A prospective crossover study of sex steroid administration in the surgical menopause." *Psychosomatic Medicine,* 474:339–351, 1985.

Tannen, D. *You Just Don't Understand: Women and Men in Conversation.* New York: Ballantine, 1991.

Tavris, C. *Anger: The Misunderstood Emotion.* New York: Touchstone, 1989.

Chapter 5

Alexandersen, P., A. Toussaint, C. Christiansen, J-P. Devagelaer et al. "Ipriflavone in the treatment of postmenopausal osteoporosis: A randomized controlled trial." *Journal of the American Medical Association* 285(11): 1482–1488, 2001.

Cawood, E.H.H. and J. Bancroft. "Steroid hormones, the menopause, sexuality and well-being of women." *Journal of Psychologic Medicine* 26:925–926, 1996.

Colditz, G.A., S.E. Hankson, D.J. Hunter, et al. "The use of estrogens and progestins and the risk of breast cancer in postmenopausal women." *New England Journal of Medicine,* 322:1589–1593, 1995.

Collaborative Group on Hormonal Factors in Breast Cancer. "Breast cancer and hormone replacement therapy: collaborative re-analysis of data from 51 epidemiological studies of 52,705 women with breast cancer and 108,411 women without breast cancer." *Lancet* 350:1047–1059, 1997.

Cooper, A., C. Spencer, M.I. Whitehead et al. "Systemic absorption of progesterone from Progest [sic] cream in postmenopausal women." *Lancet:* 351, 1998.

Darling, G.M., J.A. Johns, P.I. McCloud, S.R. Davis. "Estrogen and progestin compared with simvastatin for hypercholesteremia in postmenopausal women." *New England Journal of Medicine* 337:595–601, 1997.

Dejanikus, T. "Major drug manufacturer funds osteoporosis public education campaign." *The National Women's Health Network News,* May/June 1985.

Grodstein, F., M.J. Stampfer, G.A. Colditz et al. "Postmenopausal hormone therapy and mortality." *New England Journal of Medicine* 336(25):1769–1775, 1997.

Hulley, S., D. Grady, T. Bush et al. "Randomized trial of estrogen plus progestin for secondary prevention of coronary heart disease in post-

menopausal women: Heart & Estrogen/progestin Replacement Study
(HERS) Research Group." *Journal of the American Medical Association*
280(7); 605–613, 1998.

Jensen, J., C. Christiansen, and P. Rodbro. "Cigarette smoking, serum estrogens and bone loss during hormone replacement therapy early after
menopause." *New England Journal of Medicine, 313*(16), October 17,
1985.

Kennedy, D.L., et al. "Noncontraceptive estrogens and progestins: Use patterns over time." *Obstetrics and Gynecology, 65*(3), 441–446, 1985.

Laan, E. & R.H.W. van Lunsen. "Hormones and sexuality in postmenopausal
women." *Journal of Psychosomatic Obstetrics and Gynecology* 18:126–133,
1997.

Lee, John & Virginia Hopkins. *What Your Doctor May Not Tell You About
Menopause: The Breakthrough Book On Natural Progesterone.* Warner
Books, May 1996.

Leff, M., ed. "Do triglyceride measurements mean anything?" *Consumer
Reports on Health,* 4(8):59–60, August 1992.

Leonetti, H.B., S. Longo and J.N. Anasti. "Transdermal progesterone cream
for vasomotor symptoms and postmenopausal bone loss." *Obstetrics and
Gynecology* 94(2):225–228, 1999.

Lindsay, R. "How calcium and estrogen combine to prevent osteoporosis."
Contemporary Obstetrics and Gynecology, 27(4):108–119, April 1986.

Lucisano, A., et al. "Ovarian and peripheral androgen and estrogen levels in
postmenopausal women: Correlations with ovarian histology." *Maturitas,*
8, 1986.

Magnusson, C., J.A. Baron, N. Correia et al. "Breast cancer risk following
long-term oestrogen and oestrogen-progestin replacement therapy."
International Journal of Cancer 81:339–344, 1999.

Rako, Susan. *The Hormone of Desire: The Truth About Sexuality, Menopause
and Testosterone.* Three Rivers, 1999.

Reed, M.J., et al. "Estrogen production and metabolism in perimenopausal
women." *Maturitas,* 8, 1986.

Rodriguez, C., E.E. Calle, R.J. Coates, et al. "Estrogen replacement therapy
and fatal ovarian cancer." *American Journal of Epidemiology, 141*:828–835,
1995.

Schiff, I. "Estrogen replacement at menopause." *Harvard Medical School Health
Letter,* 12(1), November 1986.

Shapiro, S., et al. "Risk of localized and widespread endometrial cancer in
relation to recent and discontinued use of conjugated estrogens." *New
England Journal of Medicine, 313*(916), October 17, 1985.

Shipley, C.F., C.L. Simmons, and G.H. Nelson. "Comparison of transvaginal
sonography with endometrial biopsy in asymptomatic postmenopausal
women." *Journal of Ultrasound Medicine,* 13:99–104, 1994.

Sturtridge, W.C. "Osteoporosis: Its assessment, investigation, treatment and
prevention." *Geriatric Medicine,* 1, October 1985.

Wright, Jonathan V. and John Morgenthaler. *Natural Hormone Replacement for
Women Over 45.* Smart Publications, 1997.

The Writing Group for the PEPI Trial. "Effects of estrogen or estrogen/progestin regimens on heart disease risk factors in postmenopausal women." *Journal of the American Medical Association, 273*:199–208, 1995.

Chapter 6

Albers, M.M. "Osteoporosis: A health care issue for women." *Health Care for Women International*, 11:11–19 (1990).

Berkowitz, G.S., et al. "Estrogen replacement therapy and fibrocystic breast disease in postmenopausal women." *American Journal of Epidemiology, 121*(2), 1985.

Bush, T.L., and E. Barrett-Connor. "Noncontraceptive estrogen use and cardiovascular disease." *Epidemiologic Reviews*, Johns Hopkins University School of Hygiene and Public Health, 7:80–104, 1985.

Cauley, J.A., et al. "The relationship of physical activity to high density lipoprotein cholesterol in postmenopausal women." *Journal of Chronic Disease*, 39(9):687–697, 1986.

Chesnut, C.H. III. "Methods and role of bone densitometry in the estrogen-deficient woman." In *Hormone Replacement Therapy*, Swartz, ed. Baltimore, MD: Williams and Wilkins, 1992.

Cobb, J.O. "Mammography and breast self-examination: We need both." *A Friend Indeed*, 8(6), November 1991.

———. "New hope for old bones." *A Friend Indeed*, 8(2), May 1991.

———. "The tamoxifen trials." *A Friend Indeed*, 9(5), October 1992.

———. "Where the women are." In *Comprehensive Management of Menopause*, Lorrain et al, eds. New York: Springer-Verlag, 1993.

Colditz, G.A., et al. "Menopause and the risk of coronary heart disease in women." *New England Journal of Medicine*, 316(18), April 30, 1987.

Cummings, S.R., M.C. Nevitt, W.S. Browner, et al. "Risk factors for hip fracture in white women." *New England Journal of Medicine*, 332:767–773, 1995.

Dawson-Hughes, B., et al. "A controlled trial of the effect of calcium supplementation on bone density in postmenopausal women." *New England Journal of Medicine*, 323(13):878–883, 1990.

Dawson-Hughes, B., G.E. Dallal, E.A. Krall et al. "Effect of Vitamin D supplementation on wintertime and overall bone loss in healthy postmenopausal women." *Annals of International Medicine*, 115(7):505–512, 1991.

Emond, M.J. and W. Zareba. "Prognostic value of cholesterol in women of different ages." *Journal of Women's Health* 6:295–307, 1997.

Gannon, L.R. *Menstrual Disorders and Menopause: Biological, Psychological and Cultural Research*. New York: Praeger Publishers, 1985.

Hasselbring, B. "New and improved breast self-examination." *DES Action Voice*, 32, Spring 1987.

Heaney, R. "Estrogen-calcium interactions at the menopause." Paper presented at the meetings of the North American Menopause Society, Cleveland, Ohio, September 1992.

Hreschyshyn, M.M., et al. "Effects of natural menopause, hysterectomy, and oophorectomy on lumbar spine and femoral neck bone densities." *Obstetrics and Gynecology, 72*(4), 1988.

Lapidus, L. "Ischemic heart disease, stroke, and total mortality in women: Results from a prospective population study in Gothenburg, Sweden." *Acta Medica Scandia Supplement, 219*:1–42, 1986.

Lapidus, L., et al. "Triglycerides – Main lipid risk factor for cardiovascular disease in women?" *Acta Medica Scandia, 217*:481–489, 1985.

———. "Concentrations of sex-hormone binding globulin and corticosteroid binding globulin in serum in relation to cardiovascular risk factors and to 12-year incidence of cardiovascular disease and overall mortality in postmenopausal women." *Clinical Chemistry, 32*(1):146–152, 1986.

LaRosa, J.C. "Effect of estrogen replacement therapy on lipids: Implications for cardiovascular risk." *Journal of Reproductive Medicine, 30*(10), 1985.

Leff, M., ed. "Mammograms: Crucial but fallible." *Consumer Reports On Health, 3*(12):89–91, December 1991.

Love, S. *Dr. Susan Love's Breast Book.* (3rd ed.) NY: Perseus 2000.

Lubin, F., et al. "Overweight and changes in weight throughout adult life in breast cancer etiology." *American Journal of Epidemiology, 122*(4), 1985.

Melton, L.J. III. "Epidemiology of osteoporosis: Predicting who is at risk." In *Multidisciplinary Perspectives on the Menopause.* (Annals of the New York Academy of Science, 592)295–306, 1990.

Miller A., T. To, C.J. Baines, C. Wall. Canadian National Breast Screening Study 2: 13-Year Results of a Randomized Trial in Women Aged 50–59 Years. *J Natl Cancer Inst* 92(18):1490–1499, 2000.

Nabulsi, A.A., A.R. Folsom, A. White, et al. "Association of hormone replacement therapy with various cardiovascular risk factors in postmenopausal women." *New England Journal of Medicine, 328*:1069–1075, 1993.

Napoli, M.A. "New study questions breast cancer detection tests for young women but finds value to those over 50." *HealthFacts*, July 1987.

Notelovitz, M. "Exercise and health maintenance in menopausal women." In *Multidisciplinary Perspectives on the Menopause.* (Annals of the New York Academy of Science, 592)204–220, 1990.

Pak, C.Y.C., K. Sakhaee, B. Adams-Huet, et al. "Treatment of postmenopausal osteoporosis with slow-release sodium fluoride." *Annals of Internal Medicine, 123*:401–408, 1995.

Pick, R. "Atherosclerosis: The risk factors for women." *The Female Patient,* 2:60–71, 1986.

Posthuma, W.F.M., R.G.J. Westendorp, and J.P Vandebroucke. "Cardioprotective effect of hormone replacement therapy in postmenopausal women: Is the evidence biased?" *British Medical Journal,* 3089:1268–69, 1994.

Prince, R.L., et al. "Prevention of postmenopausal osteoporosis." *New England Journal of Medicine, 325*:1189–1195, 1991.

Prior, J.C., et al. "Spinal bone loss and ovulatory disturbances." *New England Journal of Medicine, 323*:1221–1227, 1990.

Richelson, L.S., et al. "Relative contributions of aging and estrogen deficiency to postmenopausal bone loss." *New England Journal of Medicine*, 311:1273–1275, 1990.

Rosen, C.F., M.F. Holick, and P.S. Millard. "Premature graying of hair is a risk marker for osteopenia." *Journal of Clinical Endocrinology and Metabolism*, 79:854–857, 1994.

Sartoris, D.J., et al. "Progress in radiology: Dual-energy radiographic absorptiometry for bone densitometry." In *Multidisciplinary Perspectives on the Menopause* (Annals of the New York Academy of Science, 592) 307–325, 1990.

Schneider, D.L., E. Barrett-Connor, and D. Morton. "Thyroid hormone use and bone mineral density in elderly women." *Journal of the American Medical Association*, 1271:1245–1249, 1994.

Sherman, B., R. Wallace, and J. Bean. "Estrogen use and breast cancer: Interaction with body mass." *Cancer*, 51:1527–1531, 1983.

Silverstolpe, G., and N. Crona. "Hormonal replacement therapy – cardiovascular disease," *Acta Obstetrics and Gynecology Scandia Supplement*, 134:93–95, 1986.

Stampfer, M.J., G.A. Colditz, W.C. Willett et al. "Postmenopausal estrogen therapy and cardiovascular disease – 10-year follow-up from the Nurses' Health Study." *New England Journal of Medicine*, 325:756–762, 1991.

Stomper, P.C., V.J. Van Voorhis, V.A. Ravnikar, and J.E. Meyer. "Mammographic changes associated with postmenopausal hormone replacement therapy: A longitudinal study." *Radiology*, 174(2):487–490, 1990.

Vandenbrouke, J.P. "Postmenopausal estrogen and cardioprotection." *Lancet*, 337:833–834, 1991.

Walsh, B.W, I. Schiff, B. Rosner et al. "Effects of postmenopausal estrogen replacement on the concentrations and metabolism of plasma lipoproteins." *New England Journal of Medicine*, 325:1196–1204, 1991.

Watts, N.B., et al. "Intermittent cyclical etidronate treatment of postmenopausal osteoporosis." *New England Journal of Medicine*, 323:73–79, 1990.

Wingo, P.A., et al. "The risk of breast cancer in postmenopausal women who have used ERT." *Journal of the American Medical Association*, 257:209–215, 1987.

Chapter 7

Aitken, J.M., et al. "Osteoporosis after oophorectomy for nonmalignant disease in premenopausal women." *British Medical Journal*, May 12, 1973.

Amerikia, H., and T.N. Evans. "Ten-year review of hysterectomies: Trends, indications and risks." *American Journal of Obstetrics and Gynecology*, 134:431–437, 1979.

Ballweg, Mary Lou, and the Endometriosis Association. *Overcoming Endometriosis: New Help from the Endometriosis Association*. New York: Congdon & Weed, 1987.

Cohen, S., and R. Soloway. "The epidemiology of gallstone disease." *Gallstones*. New York: Churchill Livingstone, 1985.

Cutler, W.B. *Hysterectomy: Before and After*. New York: Harper Collins, 1990.

Freedman, E. "Hysterectomy and sexual dysfunction." *Canadian Journal of Obstetrics and Gynecology and Women's Health Care*, 4:314, 1992.

"Gallstones: Are there alternatives to surgery?" *Harvard Medical School Health Letter*, *12*(10), August 1987.

Grodstein, F., G.A. Colditz, and M.J. Stampfer. "Postmenopausal hormone use and cholecystectomy in a large prospective study." *Obstetrics and Gynecology*, 83:5–11, 1994.

"Hysterectomy as Social Process" *Women and Health*, *10*(1), Spring 1985.

Keyser, H.H. *Women under the Knife: A Gynecologist's Report on Hazardous Medicine*. New York: Warner Books, 1984.

Kikku, P., M. Gronroos et al. "Supravaginal amputation vs. hysterectomy: Effects on libido and orgasm." *Acta Obstetrica Gynecologic Scandia*, 62:147, 1983.

McPherson, K. et al. "Regional variations in the use of common surgical procedures: Within and between England and Wales, Canada, and the United States of America." *Social Sciences in Medicine*, 15A:273–288, 1981.

Napoli, M.A., ed. "An alternative to hysterectomy?" *HealthFacts*, Vol. XI, May 1986.

Napoli, M.A., ed. "Laser surgery outclassed by a newer technology." *HealthFacts*, XVII;1–5, August 1992.

Oldenhave, A., L.J.P Jaszmann, W.T.A.M. Everaerd, et al. "Hysterectomized women with ovarian conservation report more severe climacteric complaints than do normal climacteric women of similar age." *American Journal of Obstetrics & Gynecology*, 168:765–771, 1993.

Randall, T. "Loop electrosurgical excision procedures gaining acceptance for cervical intraepithelial neoplasia," *Journal of the American Medical Association*, 266(4):460–462, July 24/31, 1991.

Reidel, H.H., et al. "Ovarian failure after hysterectomy." *Journal of Reproductive Medicine*, 31:597–600, July 1986.

Richards, D.H. "A post-hysterectomy syndrome." *Lancet*, October 26, 1974.

Roopnarinsingh, S., and T. Gopeesingh. "Hysterectomy and its psychological aftermath." *West Indian Medical Journal* 31:131, 1982.

Shainwald, S. "A legal response to hysterectomy abuse." *The National Women's Health Network News*, May/June 1985.

Simon, J.A., and G.S. diZerega. "Physiologic estradiol replacement following oophorectomy: Failure to maintain precastration gonadotropin levels." *Obstetrics and Gynecology*, 59(4), April 1982.

Stokes, N.M. *The Castrated Woman*. Toronto: Franklin Watts, 1986.

Tangedahl, T.N. "Therapeutic options for gallstones." *Postgraduate Medicine*, 81(1), January 1987.

Weinstein, K. *Living with Endometriosis: How to Cope with the Physical and Emotional Challenges*. Reading, MA: Addison-Wesley, 1987.

Weiss, N.S., and B.L. Harlow. "Why does hysterectomy without bilateral oophorectomy influence the subsequent incidence of ovarian cancer?" *American Journal of Epidemiology*, 124(5), November 1986.

Chapter 8

Brody, J.E. "Exercise is the fountain of youth." *New York Times*, June 10–11, 1986.

Council for Responsible Nutrition. *Vitamin & Mineral Safety*. Available for $10US from CRN, 1875 Eye Street N.W., Suite 400, Washington, D.C. 20006. Tel: 202-872-1488. or <www.crnusa.org/2publications.html>

"Focus on Physical Activity." *The Melpomene Report*, October 1985.

Frisch, R.E., et al. "Lower prevalence of breast cancer and cancers of the reproductive system among former college athletes compared to non-athletes." *British Journal Cancer*, 52(5):885,1985.

Health and Welfare Canada. *Nutrition Recommendations: The Report of the Scientific Review Committee*. Ottawa: Minister of Supply and Services Canada, 1990.

Lock, M., ed. "Anthropological approaches to menopause: Questioning received wisdom." *Culture, Medicine and Psychiatry*, 10(1), March 1986.

Messina, M., V. Messina, and K. Setchell. *The Simple Soybean and Your Health*. Garden City Park, NY: Avery Publishing, 1994.

Mindell, E. *Earl Mindell's Vitamin Bible for the 21st Century*. Warner Books, 1999.

Pritikin, N., and P.M. McGrady, Jr. *The Pritikin Program for Diet and Exercise*. New York: Bantam Books, 1979.

Rapport, a newsletter of the National Institute of Nutrition, 265 Carling Avenue, Suite 302, Ottawa, Ontario K1S 2E1.

Shephard, R.J. "Exercise and the aging process: Prescribing a programme." *Geriatric Medicine*, 1, October 1985.

Walsh, B.W, I. Schiff, B. Rosner et al. "Effects of postmenopausal estrogen replacement on the concentrations and metabolism of plasma lipoproteins." *New England Journal of Medicine*, 325:1196–1204, 1991.

Chapter 9

Angier, N. "Is there a male menopause? Jury is still out." *New York Times*, May 20, 1992.

Blakeslee, S. "Men's test scores linked to hormone." *New York Times*, November 14, 1991.

Brody, E.W., et al. "Women's changing roles and help to elderly parents: Attitudes of three generations of women." *Journal of Gerontology*, 38(5), September 1983.

Doering, C.H., et al. "A cycle of plasma testosterone in the human male." *Journal of Clinical Endocrinology and Metabolism*, 40:492, 1975.

Eichenbaum, L., and S. Orbach. *What Do Women Want?* New York: Berkley Pub. Grp., 1999.

Horowitz, A. "Sons and daughters as caregivers to older parents: Differences in role performance and consequences." *The Gerontologist*, 25(6), December 1985.

Lang, A.M., and E.M. Brody. "Characteristics of middle-aged daughters and help to their elderly mothers." *Journal of Marriage and the Family*, 45(1), February 1983.

Lear, M.W. "Is there a male menopause?" *New York Times Magazine*, January 28, 1973.

Lehrman, S. "Human growth hormone: The fountain of youth?" *Harvard Health Letter*, *17*(8), June 1992.

Levinson, D.J., et al. *The Seasons of a Man's Life*. New York: Harper Collins, 1990.

McKinlay, J.B., C. Longcope, and A. Gray. "The questionable physiologic and epidemiologic basis for a male climacteric syndrome: Preliminary results from the Massachusetts Male Aging Study." *Maturitas*, 11:103–115, 1989.

Morris, V., and R. Butler. *How to Care for Aging Parents*. Workman Publishing, 1996.

Moss, M.S. "The quality of relationships between elderly parents and their out-of-town children." *The Gerontologist*, *25*(2), April 1985.

Rosenthal, C.J. "Family supports in later life: Does ethnicity make a difference?" *The Gerontologist*, *26*(1), February 1986.

Rubin, L.B. *Intimate Strangers: Men and Women Together*. New York: Harper Collins, 1990.

Chapter 10

Baucer, D.C., D. Grady, and A. Pressman. "Skin thickness, estrogen use, and bone mass in older women." *Menopause: The Journal of the North American Menopause Society*, 1:131–136, 1994.

Berkun, C.S. "Changing appearance for women in the mid-years of life: Trauma?" In *Older Women: Issues and Prospects*, Markson, ed. Lexington, MA: Lexington Books, 1983.

Chernin, K. *The Obsession: Reflections on the Tyranny of Slenderness*. New York: Harper Perennial Library, 1994.

Cobb, J.O. "Male Menopause." *A Friend Indeed*, 11(4), 1994.

Fairhurst, E. "Mutton dressed as lamb: The social construction of aging." Paper presented at the 1st International Conference on the Future of Adult Life, Noordwijkerhout, The Netherlands, April 1987.

Le Guin, U.K. "On menopause: The space crone." *Medical Self Care*, Winter 1981.

Sontag, S. "The Double Standard of Aging." *Saturday Review*: 182–190, Sept. 23, 1972.

Stehlin, D. "Erasing wrinkles: Easier said than done." *FDA Consumer*, July/August 1987.

WHERE TO FIND
OR GET HELP

Today there are many more resources available for the menopausal woman than there were ten or even five years ago. More general information on the subject of menopause is available in books, booklets, newspaper and magazine articles, films, and radio and television programs. There are also many organizations that offer information on particular aspects of menopause. Many of these resources are listed following this appendix.

When you read one book, you may think you have found all that you need to know. If you read two, you are likely to find such diametrically opposed points of view that you will be compelled to read a third! If your local public or school library does not have a book you are looking for, it is worth requesting it. Menopause is a subject of interest to growing numbers of people, and most libraries are willing to order a book for you.

In addition, many organizations produce printed materials dealing with the more general aspects of menopause or with specific problems that may be more troublesome to you (migraines, hysterectomies, etc.) Much of this material is free or available at low cost. You can obtain more information by writing to or calling the particular organization, or you can contact a local woman's health organization or woman's center. They will be glad to help you find resources to fit your needs.

Menopause Clinics

Some hospitals, particularly teaching hospitals in large centers, have menopause clinics. When a woman calls me with a list of debilitating complaints and nowhere to go, I may suggest that she contact a local menopause clinic. It is not advice that I give lightly.

First of all, most women will not need the medical support of a clinic if they are seeing a doctor regularly. What they *may* need is a more understanding doctor, but the time to shop for a good doctor is before you need one. If you are not satisfied with your present doctor and you are approaching menopause, it is a good idea to ask around and get the names of three likely doctors, then make an appointment to see each in turn. If you are not experiencing any problems associated with menopause, you probably won't need to consult a doctor. But if you have a good doctor, you may not need a menopause clinic.

My basic quarrel with the menopause clinic is the confusion about its function. The main goal of a menopause clinic is *understood* by the general public to be the welfare and well-being of menopausal women. However, the primary goal of many menopause clinics is to provide data for menopausal research; helping women is secondary. Menopause clinics are usually subsidized (and supplied) by pharmaceutical companies. This means that whether you know it or not the "solutions" found for you may fall within the restricted purpose of the current research study or studies. Most of these clinics have long waiting lists, and when you finally get an appointment, you may find that you are given a certain type of drug so that the doctor can report on its effectiveness, or you may be told that you are to take a certain drug when, in fact, you have been given a placebo – a substance that looks like the product being tested but that has no effects.

There is nothing inherently wrong in this. Because of the low priority given to funding of research into women's health – a situation that is changing, I am glad to say – most hospitals *must* accept funding (and drugs) in order to continue their work. However, there is a fundamental difference between a menopause clinic and a menopause research project, and I believe this should be made clear to the women who attend. Many women go to a menopause clinic expecting individualized attention to their particular complaints, answers to their questions, and information about a range of possible treatments. This is an understandable expectation, given that their own doctors may be unprepared to deal with concerns about menopause. What these women may get instead is routine treatment as specified by the particular study under way – perhaps a general medical checkup, a short meeting with a psychologist, a short meeting with a dietitian, medication, and another appointment.

If medication is prescribed (or administered), this too will conform to whatever is being studied in that particular project. It may be an estrogen-androgen product, an estrogen tablet, a progestin tablet, or a placebo masquerading as any of these. The research study will be geared toward a particular type of drug, so that treatment varies from clinic to clinic, because the study (and the particular drug involved) will be tied to the funding of one pharmaceutical company. In other words, the menopause clinic's solution to most menopausal ailments will be a hormone preparation or two. Rarely is there familiarity with the full range of hormone and non-hormonal products available to respond to the highly individual nature of a woman's complaints.

Some clinics do get involved in studies dealing with sexuality or with psychological symptoms. If a woman is aware of the current research she will find it easier to decide whether or not to participate, and if she does, to understand and cooperate with the process. She may wish to ask for copies of the completed research papers.

Not all menopause clinics are this narrow, although I know of one that threw open its doors, welcomed patients until the study results were in, then promptly closed. Potential patients were told that it had been too popular, but the truth was that the pharmaceutical company's research funds had been withdrawn.

There may be a menopause clinic available in your community that does *not* operate in this manner. Your best bet is to inquire about sources of funding and medication provided by the clinic before you enroll.

Menopause Seminars

Hospitals, women's health centers, and service organizations (often in conjunction with hospitals) occasionally present one-time menopause seminars or information sessions. Pharmaceutical companies often sponsor such seminars, although the sponsorship is rarely publicized. These sessions, however they are labeled, usually take place in a medium to large hall (often a hospital or university auditorium) and permit very limited questions and answers from the floor. Most will feature medical experts, usually a doctor or doctors (sometimes a psychiatrist), occasionally a physiotherapist, and/or dietitian. These types of sessions often appeal to very busy women who want a quick, one-shot dose of information.

The basic problem with these kinds of sessions is that they often ignore the great diversity of opinion within the medical profession and among nonmedical researchers. What you get is one doctor's (or a few doctors') opinions about menopause, based on the women they see and the research they do. Because most doctors are faithful to a medical model of menopause (the model that views it as a "deficiency condition") and because they rarely see healthy menopausal women, what they have to say may or may not correspond with your own experience. Some women discover that specialists (gynecologists) have such divergent views on menopause that they are better off consulting their family doctors. These sessions often bolster the image of gynecologist as all-knowing and there is rarely opportunity for discussion of the very real concerns that most women harbor.

These kinds of sessions are popular with women who are reluctant to commit themselves to more than one day or one evening for learning about menopause. The problem is that they may leave more confused than ever. A better bet for those who may not wish to air their problems and who do not want to listen to the problems of others is the menopause workshop.

Menopause Workshops

The menopause workshop may also be called a discussion group or seminar, or may appear as part of the course offerings of a continuing education or adult education section of a local school, college, or university. Whatever its name, the workshop is usually scheduled at a particular time and location, to take place for a specified number of sessions, in a neutral setting. Someone trained in group work is hired to facilitate the discussion, and "experts" may be invited to some sessions to explain particular aspects of menopause. Depending on the size of the group and the topics to be covered, there may or may not be ample opportunity to air individual concerns.

The atmosphere in this kind of group depends on the continuing presence of a core group, the duration of the sessions, the number of sessions, how the women interact with one another, and the skills of the facilitator in putting people at ease. It is difficult to predict how satisfying the workshop will be for the individual participant, but the increased demand for such workshops across the country is testimony to their success.

These kinds of workshops should not be confused with the one-shot workshop that is often held in conjunction with an all-day information session on women's health issues. Often, smaller groups "workshop" on particular topics as a follow-up to a more general information session in the morning.

A good workshop offers both structured information and moral support – both contribute to the sense that one's menopausal experiences are *not* unique, that one *can* cope, and that menopause is but a temporary disruption. If the structure of an ongoing workshop appeals to you, it may be worth your while to contact some appropriate agencies in your community (your church or synagogue, school boards, community college, women's organization, YWCA, etc.). Often a call is enough to get the ball rolling.

Many women who have attended workshops or discussion groups become so involved with the whole process of group learning that they are inspired to become trained facilitators themselves. Many community women's organizations both encourage and enable their members to learn the skills of facilitating groups, either in courses that they develop themselves or through programs at local colleges or universities.

Some women live too far away from the kinds of institutions that are likely to sponsor menopause workshops. Some women like the idea of the moral support, but are not particularly interested in a review of the physiological processes of menopause and are daunted by the thought of a large group or a classroom. Some women would rather attend sessions at a different time of day, and may be interested in the more informal, often more intimate self-help group (also known as a mutual aid group or support group).

Self-Help Groups

Self-help groups are formed because the people in them are (or will be) experiencing something in common and because they want to talk together to help themselves and help one another. Self-help groups are not a substitute for professional help (although they are often a valuable adjunct to professional help) and are not dependent on professional expertise. Self-help groups require a willingness to make the group work and a commitment from each member of the group to attend the first three or four meetings. Anything else can be decided once the group gets under way.

There are various opinions about the optimum size for a self-help group, but the consensus seems to be in the range of six to twelve. The smaller the group, the more reliant you will be on the commitment of the members to the group; at the same time, smaller groups often foster more intimacy more quickly. Some groups adopt an "open door" policy, encouraging new members to join the group at any time. Others prefer to encourage intimacy and trust by closing the group, either for a limited number of meetings or for the group's duration. If the decision is made to close the group, each member will have to make a solid commitment to attend.

If you wish to start a self-help group, you have various options. You can enlist the help of friends or acquaintances to find members. In other words, from the beginning, you can *share* the job of recruiting. If word of mouth is inadequate, you might consider advertising – posting a notice on a bulletin board, placing an ad in a community newspaper or a church bulletin, etc. Your doctor or your friends' doctors may be willing to help by mentioning the idea to likely patients. Sometimes self-help groups can be recruited within the context of a larger meeting. Perhaps an existing women's group will agree to show a film on menopause, or a local organization may be willing to sponsor a presentation about menopause. This provides an opportunity to ask women who attend to sign up if they're interested in a self-help group, or to circulate a "sign-in" sheet and then contact each woman by telephone to see if she (and/or a friend) would be interested in joining the group.

The decision about where to hold the meetings is often a difficult one. The first meeting should be held in a "neutral" place – a school, library, community center, church, etc. – some place that's convenient and accessible. You may decide to hold subsequent meetings in one another's homes, but this will depend on the size of the group and the living situation of the members. The meeting places should be protected from interruption from telephone calls, unexpected callers, and other family members.

No matter how you get started, the first meeting is often taken up with organizational questions. Even when *you* have a clear idea of why you wanted to start a group, you will find that others may have different ideas. It helps if you can articulate and obtain agreement about the general purpose of the group (e.g., "to help us to feel more comfortable about and with menopause"), leaving the precise ways to achieve this to be decided by the group. If the word *menopause* gets in the way of forming a group, a more acceptable goal might be "the exploration of changes in midlife" or something general and non-threatening. Widow-to-widow groups or groups for divorced women in their forties or fifties may view menopause as part of a more global objective. Whatever the goal, each member will arrive with her own "hidden agenda" – needs that may or may not be fulfilled by this particular group. In other words, although there may be consensus about the general goal of the self-help group, each person's way of achieving this is likely to be different. This is where the group must formulate specific objectives or tasks to be accomplished at each meeting.

Most self-help groups attempt to meet once a week, but you may find that once every two weeks is more convenient for your members. The meeting itself should run for at least two hours; some groups find that three hours are necessary to allow time for everyone. If coffee (decaffeinated) or herbal tea is served, this should be confined to a short period just before or just after the meeting. Some groups like to set up an agenda, with specific topics slotted for a particular evening. And, as I have said, they may also wish to limit the life of the group to a definite number of sessions. (Six is usually the minimum, but some groups aim for eight or decide to just keep things open-ended.) Other groups prefer to see how much can be covered in one meeting and to spend the last few minutes deciding on the topic for the next. This kind of group may endure for as long as the members feel a need for it.

The thousands of letters that I've received over the years since *A Friend Indeed* was founded tell me that there is one group of women who desperately need this kind of support: younger women who are dealing with an unexpected and very early menopause, either brought on by surgery or occurring naturally. If those of you who work in a women's health center could read, as I have, anguished letters from young women who feel isolated, who cannot understand their own physical and psychological reactions, who are desperate to feel sexual desire, then you would understand why this is so important. Women in their forties don't feel this sense of abandonment because they are more likely to know other women going through the same thing. But if you are in your twenties or thirties, as many women are when menopause is forced upon them, it is hard to know where to turn.

One of the greatest benefits of a group is the new sense of intimacy with women who can empathize with your experience. Yet members of self-help groups can do much more than express feelings to one another. They can choose to take action about behaviors that contribute, directly or indirectly, to each woman's well-being. Groups of midlife women can get together to exercise – take "power walks" as a group and then sit down for a meeting afterward. Or they can hire a fitness instructor and enjoy a Jazzercise or aerobics class together. Some groups might be interested in learning more about nutrition and practicing recipes based on low-fat or no-fat cooking. Such groups might be formed as a way of fostering general good health, or as a way of coping when a family member suffers from some form of cardiovascular disease. Women who house or care for dependent parents often need the aid and support of other women. A group formed around this issue may be of enormous help to other women who find themselves suddenly placed in the same situation.

Together, group members can locate and evaluate doctors in the community, even if the need for doctors' services is not imminent. If a member of the group is apprehensive about a visit to the doctor, another member of the group may go along to offer moral support. There are all sorts of possibilities for a self-help group.

Perhaps this is the greatest gift that menopause brings – the opportunity to reach out to others and to find that in helping one another, we develop resources, strengths, and abilities that we never knew we had.

References

Cobb, J.O. "How to start a menopause self-help group." *A Friend Indeed*, 4(7), December 1987.

————. "Premature menopause." *A Friend Indeed*, 8(9), February 1992.

North American Menopause Society. *How To Develop a Menopause Discussion Group*. ($15.00 U.S. plus $8.00 for shipping single copy) Available from P.O. Box 94527, Cleveland, OH 44101-4527. Website: <www.menopause.org>

GENERAL

RESOURCES

1. Books relating to women's health and/or menopause. Most are available in paperback through <www.amazon.com>.

Barbach, Lonnie G. *The Pause: a Positive Approach to Menopause* (rev. ed.). New York: Plume, 2000.

Boston Women's Health Book Collective. *Our Bodies Ourselves for the New Century*. New York: Touchstone, 1998.

Breen, Mary J., and Lindsay Hall. *So Many Changes: Women, Health and Midlife*. Toronto: Lawrence Heights Community Health Centre Press. 1999.

Brown, Susan E. *Better Bones, Better Body: A Comprehensive Self-Help Program for Preventing, Halting and Overcoming Osteoporosis*. Keats Publishing Company, 2000.

Burgio, Kathryn L., K. Lynette Pearce, and Angelo J. Lucco. *Staying Dry: A Practical Guide to Bladder Control*. Baltimore, MD: The Johns Hopkins University Press, 1990.

Cabot, Sandra. *Smart Medicine for Menopause: Hormone Replacement Therapy and Its Natural Alternatives*. New York: Penguin Putnam, 1999.

Cole, Ellen, and Esther D. Rothblum (eds.) *Women and Sex Therapy: Closing the Circle of Sexual Knowledge*. Binghamton, NY: Haworth Press, 1996.

Coney, Sandra. *The Menopause Industry: How the Medical Establishment Exploits Women*. Alameda, CA: Hunter House, 1994.

Crawford, Amanda McQuade. *The Herbal Menopause Book: Herbs, Nutrition and Other Natural Therapies*. Freedom, CA: The Crossing Press, 1996.

Crook, Marion. *My Body: Women Speak Out About Their Health Care*. New York: Plenum Publishing, 1995.

Cutler, Winnifred Berg. *Hysterectomy: Before and After*. New York: Harper Collins, 1990.

DeMarco, Carolyn. *Take Charge of Your Body* (rev. 6th ed.) Winlaw, B.C.: The Well Woman Press, 1996.

Edwards, Peggy, Miroslava Lhotsky, M.D., and Judy Turner, Ph.D. *The Healthy Boomer: A No-Nonsense Midlife Health Guide for Women and Men.* Toronto: McClelland and Stewart, 1999.

Gaby, Allan R. *Preventing and Reversing Osteoporosis.* Rocklin, CA: Prima Publishing, 1994.

Greenwood, Sadja. *Menopause Naturally* (4th ed.). San Francisco: Volcano Press, 1996.

Henkel, Gretchen, and PG Stumpf. *The Menopause Sourcebook.* Los Angeles: Lowell House, 2000.

Holmberg-Schwartz, Deborah. *Catching Our Breath: A Journal About Change for Women Who Smoke.* Winnipeg: Women's Health Clinic, 1997.

Huston, James, and L. Darlene Lanka. *Perimenopause: Changes in Women's Health After 35.* Los Angeles: Lowell House, 1997.

Hutchinson, Karen Anne, and Judith Sachs. *What Every Woman Needs To Know About Estrogen: Natural and Traditional Therapies For a Longer, Healthier Life.* New York: Plume 1997.

Lambert-Lagacé, Louise. *Good Nutrition for a Healthy Menopause.* Toronto: Stoddart Publishing, 1999.

Laux, Marcus, and Christine Conrad. *Natural Woman, Natural Menopause.* New York: Harper Collins, 1998.

Love, Susan M. (with Karen Lindsey). *Dr. Susan Love's Hormone Book: Making Informed Choices About Menopause.* New York: Random House, 1998.

Love, Susan M. (with Karen Lindsey). *Dr. Susan Love's Breast Book (3rd ed.)* New York: Perseus, 2000.

Maas, Paula, Susan E. Brown, and Nancy Bruning. *The Mend Clinic Guide to Natural Medicine for Menopause and Beyond.* New York: Dell Publishing, 1997.

McCain, Marian Van Eyk. *Transformation through Menopause.* New York: Bergin and Garvey, 1991.

Moulton, A.W., C. Landau, and M.G. Cyr. *The Complete Book of Menopause.* Berkley Publishing Group, 1995.

National Women's Health Network. *Taking Hormones and Women's Health: Choices, Risks, Benefits,* April 2000. Available for $15 (U.S. funds) from NWHN: 514 Tenth Street N.W., Suite 400, Washington, D.C., 20004. Website: <www.womenshealthnetwork.org>.

Nelson, Miriam. *Strong Women, Strong Bones.* New York: Bantam, 1999.

Northrup, Christiane. *Women's Bodies, Women's Wisdom: Creating Physical and Emotional Health and Healing* (2nd rev.). New York: Bantam Doubleday Dell, 1998.

———. *The Wisdom of Menopause: Creating Physical and Emotional Health and Healing During the Change.* New York: Bantam Doubleday Dell, 2001.

Notelovitz, Morris, and Diane Tonnessen. *Menopause & Midlife Health* (3rd ed.) New York: St. Martin's Press, 1994.

Null, Gary, and Barbara Seaman. *For Women Only! Your Guide to Health Empowerment.* New York: Seven Stories Press, 1999.

Omichinski, Linda. *You Count, Calories Don't* (2nd ed.) Portage La Prairie, MB: HUGS International, 1999. (HUGS International, Inc., Box 102A, R.R. #3, Portage La Prairie, MB R1N 3A3. Website: <www.hugs.com>.)

Page, Lafern. *Menopause and Emotions: Making Sense of Your Feelings When Your Feelings Make No Sense.* Vancouver: Primavera Press, 1993.

Perry, Susan, and Katherine O'Hanlan. *Natural Menopause: The complete guide to a woman's most misunderstood passage.* New York: Perseus, 1996.

Petras, Kathryn. *The Premature Menopause Book: When the "Change of Life" Comes Too Early.* New York: Avon Books, 1999.

Rinzler, Carol Ann. *Estrogen and Breast Cancer: A Warning to Women* (2nd ed.) New York: Hunter House, 1996.

Schiff, Isaac, and Ann B. Parsons. *Menopause: The most comprehensive, up-to-date information available to help you understand this stage of life, make the right treatment choices, and cope effectively.* New York: Times Books, 1996.

Voda, Ann M. *Menopause Me and You: The Sound of Women Pausing.* Harrington Park Press, 1997.

Weed, Susan S. *Menopausal Years: The Wise Woman Way, Alternative Approaches for Women 30 to 90.* Woodstock, N.Y.: Ash Tree Publishing, 1992.

Wolfe, Honora Lee. *Managing Menopause Naturally with Chinese Medicine.* Boulder: Blue Poppy Press, 1998. Website: <www.bluepoppy.com>.

Wright, Carol V., and Mary J. Minkin. *What Every Woman Needs To Know About Menopause: The Years, Before, During, and After.* Yale University Press, 1997

2. Booklets

Agency for Health Care Policy and Research. *Urinary Incontinence: A Patient's Guide.* AHCPR Publication #0684, March 1996. Downloadable from <http://hstat.nim.nih.gov/ftrs/tocview>.

Heart and Stroke Foundation of Canada. Women, Heart Disease, and Stroke in Canada: Issues and Options, 1997. (See listing under "Canadian organizations.")

North American Menopause Society. *Menopause, A New Beginning.* Cleveland: NAMS, 1998. (A 26-page booklet in clear language useful for women less comfortable with English or with low literacy skills. Illustrated with helpful suggestions. Best ordered in multiples by a clinic or physician.)

———. *Menopause Guidebook.* Cleveland: NAMS, 1998. (A 50-page overview of various aspects of menopause.)

———. *Induced Menopause Guidebook: When Medical Interventions Cause Menopause.* Cleveland: NAMS, 1999. (A 28-page resource for women experiencing menopause due to surgery, chemotherapy or radiation therapy.)

To order see listing under "U.S. Organizations."

3. Organizations dealing with women's health. Some publish a newsletter, some provide information, some are local organizations which run workshops or sponsor self-help groups.

a. *International organizations*

International Menopause Society, c/o Monique Boulet, Executive Director, Chez Maître M. Steyaert, Av. Des Cattleyas, 3, box 1, 1150 Brussels, Belgium. Telephone: 011 (32-2) 772-2183. Fax: 011 (32-2) 762-4295. The primary objective of the IMS is to promote the study of all aspects of the climacteric in both men and women but, in practice, the Society (which is composed primarily of gynecologists) promotes the study of medical intervention in the female menopause. It holds a Congress every third year, the next one scheduled for 2002. In addition to organizing congresses, symposia, and workshops, the IMS publishes a quarterly newsletter and also its own journal, *Climacteric, the Journal of the International Menopause Society*. Membership is $125 (U.S.) per year which includes a subscription to *Climacteric*. Website: <www.imsociety.org>.

International Academy of Compounding Pharmacists. Telephone: (800) 927-4227. Website: <www.iacprx.org>.

International Foundation for Functional Gastrointestinal Disorders (IFFGD), Box 17864, Milwaukee, WI 53217. Telephone: (414) 964-1799. Bulletin $35 (US) per year. Website: <www.iffgd.org>.

Isis International: the Latin American and Caribbean Women's Health Network, Silvina Hurtado 1864, Providencia 664067, Santiago, Chile. Also P.O. Box 1837, Quezon City, Philippines. Isis has two offices – one in Manila that focuses on the Asia-Pacific region; and another in Chile. Each office produces a regular magazine: the quarterly *Mujeres en Accion* in Spanish from the Chile office and the triannual *Women's Health Journal* in English from the Manila office. The Manila office also publishes the monthly *Women Envision*. Websites: <www.isiswomen.org> or <www.reddesalud.web.cl/ingles.html>.

Women's Global Network on Reproductive Rights, Vrolikstraat 453-D, 1092 TJ Amsterdam, The Netherlands. Telephone: 011 (31-20) 620-9672. Fax: 011 (31-20) 622-2450. Website: <www.wgnrr.org>.

Women's Health Action Foundation has salient information on drugs. Contact them by e-mail at the Wemos Foundation, P.O. Box 1693, 1000 BR Amsterdam, The Netherlands. Telephone: 011 (31-20) 468-8388. Fax: 011 (31-20) 468-6008. E-mail: <wemos@wemos.nl.>. Website: <www.wemos.nl>.

Women's Health Information Centre, 52 Featherstone Street, London, EC1, England. Membership entitles you to a newsletter, fact sheets and broadsheets published during that year. Membership is £5 for individuals. Telephone 011(44-171) 251-6580. Fax 011(44-171) 608-0928. Website: <www.womenshealthlondon.org.uk>.

b. *U.S. organizations*

Endometriosis Association, U.S./Canada Headquarters, 8585 N. 76th Place, Milwaukee, WI 53223, U.S.A., Telephone: (414) 355-2200. Fax: (414) 355-6065. Publishes regular bulletins, leaflets (e.g., "How Can I Tell If I Have Endometriosis?") and a book, *The Endometriosis Sourcebook*. The Association acts as a support network with regional chapters, support groups and crisis call volunteers. The EA will try to provide information about doctors skilled in diagnosing and treating osteoporosis. Website: <www.EndometriosisAssn.org>.

HERS (Hysterectomy Educational Resources and Services), 422 Bryn Mawr Avenue, Bala Cynwyd, PA 19004, U.S.A. Telephone (610) 667-7757. Fax (610) 667-8096. Will also supply reprints of articles on specific topics. Websites: <www.hersfoundation.com> and <www.uterinearteryembolization.com>.

The IC [Interstitial Cystitis] Network, 4773 Sonoma Highway, Suite 235, Santa Rosa, CA 95409. Telephone: (707) 538-9442. Website: <www.sonic.net/jill/icnet>

Interstitial Cystitis Association of America, Inc., 51 Monroe St., Suite 1402, Rockville, MD 20850. Telephone: (301) 610-5300. Website: <www.ichelp.org>

Intestinal Disease Foundation (IDF), 1323 Forbes Ave., Suite 200, Pittsburgh, PA 15219. Telephone: (412) 261-5888.

Melpomene Institute for Women's Health Research, 1010 University Avenue, St. Paul, MN 55104. Telephone: (651) 642-1951. Fax: (651) 642-1951. Sponsors research on women's health with a special interest in exercise, occasional weekend seminars on a variety of topics, and the *Melpomene Journal* (see Newsletters and Periodicals). Website: <www.melpomene.org>.

National Association for Continence (NAFC), Box 8310, Spartanburg, SC 29305. Telephone: (800) 252-3337 or (864) 579-7900. Fax: (864) 579-7902. Publishes a quarterly newsletter, which is free with a $15 (US) membership fee, and a *Resource Guide of Continence Aids and Services*. Website: <www.nafc.org>.

National Fibromyalgia Partnership, 140 Zinn Way, Linden, VA 22642-5609. Telephone: (866) 725-4404 or (540) 622-2998. E-mail: <mail@fmpartnership.org>. Website: <www.fmpartnership.org>. Another source of information about fibromyalgia is <www.mayoclinic.com/home?id=DS00079>.

National Lymphedema Network (NLN), Latham Square, 1611 Telegraph Avenue, Suite 1111, Oakland, CA 94612-2138. Pamphlets and books available from NLN online shopping page. Telephone: (800) 541-3259 or (510) 208-320. Fax: (510) 208-3110. Website: <www.lymphnet.org>.

National Vulvodynia Association, P.O. Box 4491, Silver Spring, MD 20914-4491. Membership is $40 (US) a year and entitles members to a quarterly newsletter, a bibliography of relevant articles and, if desired, a confidential share list. Telephone: (941) 927-8503. Fax: (941) 927-8602. Website: <www.nva.org>.

National Women's Health Network, 514 Tenth Street N.W., Suite 400, Washington, D.C., 20004. Telephone: (202) 628-7814. Fax: (202) 347-1168. [The NWHN provides information packets containing a glossary, resource list, 3-5 articles and an extensive annotated bibliography on a range of issues dealing with women's health. Packets are $8 (US) each.] Membership is $25 (US) per year for individuals. Website: <www.womenshealthnetwork. org>.

North American Menopause Society, P.O. Box 94527, Cleveland, OH 44101-4527. Telephone: (440) 442-7550. Members [$170 (US) annually] are entitled to the quarterly journal *Menopause*, as well as the publication *Menopause Management* and the newsletter *Flashes*. NAMS meets annually in various North American cities. Website: <www.menopause.org>.

Osteoporosis Education Project and the Nutrition Education and Consulting Service, 605 Franklin Park Drive, East Syracuse, NY 13057. Provides detailed information about bone health and nutrients. Telephone: (315) 432-9231. Fax: (315) 463-7706. Website: <www.betterbones.com>.

Premature Ovarian Failure (POF) Support Group, P.O. Box 23643, Alexandria, VA 22304. Membership is $25(US) a year which includes a quarterly newsletter, a referral list of health care providers, and a confidential share list. Website: <www.pofsupport.org>.

Restless Leg Syndrome Foundation, P.O. Box 314-JH, 514 Daniels St., Raleigh, NC 27605. Members $30(US) includes the quarterly newsletter, *Night Walkers*, as well as medical bulletins and a bibliography that can be mailed directly to your physician. Website: <www.ris.org>.

Society for Menstrual Cycle Research, c/o Mary Anna Friederich, M.D., 10559 North 104th Place, Scottsdale, AZ 85258. Membership [$35 (US) or $15 for students] comprises a quarterly newsletter, news about bi-annual meetings, and participation in a members' listserver. Website: <www.pop.psu.edu/smcr>.

Vulvar Pain Foundation, Drawer 177, 433 Ward St., Graham, NC 27253. Membership is $45(US) per year, entitling you to the newsletter, and other benefits. Website: <www.vulvarpainfoundation.org>.

Women's International Pharmacy, 5708 Monona Drive, Madison, WI 53716. Telephone (800) 279-5708 or (623) 714-7700. Fax: (800) 279-8011. Also 13925 West Meeker Blvd., Suite 13, Sun City West, AZ 85375. Telephone: (800) 699-8144 or (608) 221-7800. Fax: (800) 613-8862. Website: <www.womensinternational.com>.

c. *Canadian organizations*

Aboriginal Nurses Association, 12 Stirling Avenue, 3rd floor, Ottawa, ON K1Y 1P8. Telephone: (613) 724-4677. Fax: (613) 724-4718. Website: <www.anac.on.ca>.

Access Alliance Multicultural Community Health Centre, 509 College Street, Toronto On M6G 1A8.

ACCÉSSS (Alliance des communautés culturelles pour l'égalité dans la santé et les services sociaux), 1030 rue Beaubien est, Bureau 301, Montréal, QC H2S 1T4.

Allergy/Asthma Information Association, Box 100, Toronto, ON M9W 5K9. Telephone: (800) 611-7011 or (416) 679-9521. Fax: (416) 670-9524. Website: <www.aaia.ca>.

Alzheimer Society of Canada, 20 Eglinton Avenue, West, Suite 1200, Toronto, ON M4R 1K8. Telephone: (800) 616-8816 or (416) 488-8772. Fax: (416) 488-3778. Website: <www.alzheimer.ca>.

The Arthritis Society, 393 University Avenue, Suite 1700, Toronto, ON M5G 1E6. Telephone: (800) 321-1433 or (416) 979-7228. Fax: (416) 979-8366. Regional offices in St. John's, Charlottetown, Halifax, Fredericton, Montreal, Winnipeg, Regina, Calgary and Vancouver. Website: <www.arthritis.ca>.

Association canadienne des femmes arabes, 5560 rue Casgrain, Montreal, QC H2T 1X9.

Association of Specialists in Plastic and Cosmetic Surgery of Quebec, 2 Complexe Desjardins, C.P. 216, Succursale Complexe Desjardins, Montreal, QC H5B 1G8. Telephone: (514) 350-5109. Fax: (514) 350-5151.

Association of Women of India in Canada, 3030 Don Mills Road East, Suite LL8A11, North York, ON M2J 3C1.

Asthma Society of Canada, 130 Bridgeland Avenue, Suite 425, Toronto, ON M6A 1Z4. Telephone: (800) 787-3880 or (416) 787-4050. Fax: (416) 787-5807.

Canadian Academy of Facial Plastic and Reconstructive Surgeons, c/o Mount Sinai Hospital, 600 University Avenue, Room 401, Toronto, ON M5G 1X5. Telephone: (416) 569-6965. Fax: (905) 569-6960.

Canadian Alopecia Areata Association, P.O. Box 42084, R.P.O. Millbourne, Edmonton, AB T6K 4C4. Telephone: (403) 486-6343.

Canadian Association on Gerontology, 824 Meach Street, Suite 100, Ottawa, ON K1Z 6E8. Telephone: (613) 728-9347. Fax: (613) 728-8913. Website: <www.cagacg.ca>.

Canadian Breast Cancer Foundation, 790 Bay Street, Suite 1000, Toronto, ON M5G 1N8. Telephone: (800) 387-9816 or (416) 596-6773. Fax: (416) 596-7857. Website: <www.cbcf.org>.

Canadian Cancer Society, 10 Alcorn Avenue, Suite 200, Toronto, ON M4V 3B1. Telephone: (416) 961-7223. Fax: (416) 961-4189. Website: <www.cancer.ca>.

Canadian Cardiovascular Society, 222 Queen Street, Suite 1403, Ottawa, ON K1P 5V9. Telephone: (613) 569-3407. Fax: (613) 569-6574. Website: <www.ccs.ca>.

Canadian Chinese Women's Association, 5849 University Avenue, Halifax, NS B3H 4H7.

Canadian College of Naturopathic Medicine, 1255 Sheppard Avenue East, Toronto, ON M2K 1E2. Telephone: (416) 498-1255. Fax: (416) 498-1576. A training facility for practitioners of naturopathy. Website: <www.ccnm.edu>.

Canadian Congress on Learning Opportunities for Women (CCLOW), 256 Jarvis Street, Suite 5A, Toronto, ON M5B 2J4. Telephone: (416)

599-2854. Fax: (416) 599-5605. Networks in all provinces and territories. CCLOW is a national organization that promotes feminist education and the empowerment of women. Membership is $30 (students $10). Website: <www.nald.ca/cclow.htm>.

Canadian Council of Muslim Women, 513–2400 Dundas Street, Toronto, ON L5K 2R8.

Canadian Dermatology Foundation, 450 Central Avenue, Suite 309, London, ON N6B 2E8. Telephone: (519) 432-3968. Fax: (519) 673-4666. Website: <www.cdf.ca>.

Canadian Diabetes Association, 15 Toronto Street, Suite 800, Toronto, ON M5C 2E3. Telephone: (416) 363-3373. Fax: (416) 363-3393.

Canadian Health Coalition, c/o Mike McBane, 2841 Riverside Drive, Ottawa, ON K1V 8X7. Telephone: (613) 521-3400, Extension 308. This is a group formed to educate the general public about threats to the medicare system. Website: <www.healthcoalition.ca>.

Canadian Interstitial Cystitis Society (CICS), Attn: Sandy McNicol (President), P.O. Box 28625, 4050 East Hastings Street, Burnaby, BC V5C 2H0. Telephone: (250) 758-3207. Fax: (250) 758-4894.

Canadian Mental Health Association, 2160 Yonge Street, 3rd Floor, Toronto, ON M4S 2Z3. Telephone: (416) 484-7750. Fax: (416) 484-4617. Website: <www.cmha.ca>.

Canadian Public Health Association, 1565 Carling Avenue, Suite 400, Ottawa, ON K1Z 8R1. Telephone: (613) 725-3769. Fax: (613) 725-9826. Non-profit organization seeking to improve personal and community health. Website: <www.cpha.ca/english/index.htm>.

Canadian Research Institute for the Advancement of Women (CRIAW), 151 Slater Street, Suite 408, Ottawa, ON K1P 5H3. Telephone: (613) 563-0681. Fax: (613) 563-0682. Encourages, promotes and disseminates research into women's experience. Publishes a newsletter, *The CRIAW Papers*, and *Feminist Perspectives*. Website: <www.criaw-icref.ca>.

Canadian Society of Esthetic Plastic Surgery. Will provide names of accredited plastic surgeons in your area. Telephone: (800) 263-4429. Fax: (905) 831-7248. Website: <www.csaps.ca>.

Canadian Women's Health Network, 419 Graham Avenue, Suite 203, Winnipeg, MB R3C 0M3. Telephone: (204) 942-5500. Fax: (204) 989-2355. A bilingual network linking individuals, groups and organizations concerned with women's health across Canada. The CWHN provides access to health information, health policies and research relevant to women of all ages through databases, a toll-free number and its quarterly newsletter, *Network/Le Réseau*. E-mail: <cwhn@cwhn.ca>. Website: <www.cwhn.ca>.

Centres of Excellence for Women's Health Program, Women's Health Bureau, Health Canada, 3rd floor, Jeanne Mance Building – 1903C, Tunney's Pasture, Ottawa, ON K1A 0K9. Telephone (613) 952-0765. Funded by Health Canada, five Centres of Excellence produce policy-relevant research on issues related to women's health, involving academics, health care providers and community groups in research partnerships. The

Canadian Women's Health Network (see above) coordinates networking and communication for the CEWH Program. E-mail: <cewhp@hc-sc.gc.ca>. Website: <www.hc-sc.gc.ca/women>.

Congress of Black Women of Canada (Ottawa Chapter), 1605–1535 Alta Vista Drive, Ottawa, ON K1G 3N9. Website: <www.geocities.com/Wellesley/Gazebo/8420/congress_of_black_women. htm>.

Crohn's and Colitis Foundation of Canada, 21 St. Clair Avenue East, Suite 301, Toronto, ON M4T 1L9. Telephone: (416) 920-5035. Fax: (416) 929-0364. Members receive the quarterly CRIC Journal. Website: <www.ccfc.ca>.

DAWN (Disabled Women's Network). A national organization controlled by and comprised of disabled women. 140 Elliot Avenue, Suite 102, Kingston, ON K76 6P1. Telephone: (613) 546-7387. Fax: (613) 546-7387, or P.O. Box 22003, Downtown P.O., Brandon, MB R7A 6Y9. Telephone: (204) 726-1406. Fax: (204) 726-1409. Website: <dawncanada.net>.

DES Action/Canada, P.O. Box 233, Snowdon Station, Montreal, PQ H3X 3T4. Telephone: (514) 482-3204. Providing information about DES (diethylstilbestrol), a synthetic estrogen prescribed between 1941 and 1971 to prevent miscarriage and which caused health problems in many daughters and sons as well as in mothers who took the drug. Publishes a quarterly newsletter about DES and other related drug safety issues, and can put you in touch with your local representatives. DES Action USA also publishes a newsletter, DES Action Voice. Website: <www.web.net/~desact>.

Dietitians of Canada, 480 University Avenue, Suite 604, Toronto, ON M5G 1V2. Telephone: (416) 596-0857. Fax: (416) 596-0603. Website: <www.dietitians.ca>.

Heart and Stroke Foundation. Head Office, 222 Queen Street, Suite 1402, Ottawa, ON K1P 5V9. Telephone: (613) 569-4361. Fax: (613) 569-3278. Website: <www.heartandstroke.ca>.

Infertility Awareness Association of Canada, 1 Nicholas Street, Suite 406, Ottawa, ON K1N 7B7. Telephone: (613) 244-7222 or (800) 263-2929. Website: <www.iaac.ca>.

Lesbian Mothers Support Society, P.O. Box 61, Station M, Calgary, AB T2P 2G9. Telephone: (403) 265-6433. Website: <www.lesbian.org/lesbian.moms>.

Metis National Council of Women, Inc. 1 Nicholas Street, Suite 500, Ottawa, ON K1N 7B7.

The Migraine Foundation, 365 Bloor Street, East, Suite 1912, Toronto, ON M4W 3L4. Telephone: (800) 663-3557 or (416) 920-4916. Fax: (416) 920-3577. Website: <www.migraine.ca>.

Multiple Sclerosis Society of Canada, 250 Bloor Street East, Suite 1000, Toronto, ON M4W 3P9. Telephone: (416) 922-6065, or (800) 268-7582. Fax: (416) 922-7538. Website: <www.mssociety.ca>.

National Action Committee on the Status of Women, Health Committee, 234 Eglinton Avenue East, Suite 203, Toronto, ON M4P 1K5.

Telephone: (416) 932-1718. Fax: (416) 932-0646. NAC is a voluntary, feminist, non-governmental organization and represents over 700 non-governmental women's groups. Website: <www.nac-cca.ca>.

National Cancer Institute of Canada, 10 Alcorn Avenue, Suite 200, Toronto, ON M4V 3B1. Telephone: (416) 961-7223. Fax: (416) 961-7327. (See also Canadian Cancer Society.) Website: <www.ncic.cancer.ca>.

National Organization of Immigrant and Visible Minority Women in Canada, 251 Bank Street, Suite 504, Ottawa, ON K2P 1X3.

Native Women's Association of Canada, 9 Melrose Avenue, Ottawa, ON K1Y 1T8.

Native Women's Resource Centre, 191 Gerrard Street East, Toronto, ON M5A 2E5.

North American Chronic Pain Association of Canada, 150 Central Park Drive, Suite 105, Brampton, ON L6T 2T9. Telephone: (800) 616-PAIN or (905) 793-4230. Fax: (905) 793-8781. Website: <www.chronicpaincanada.org>.

One Voice, The Canadian Seniors Network, 12 Eddy Street, Suite 100, Hull QC J8X 2W5. Telephone: (888) 867-1111 or (819) 770-3131. Fax: (819) 770-5833. A lobbying organization for seniors. Website: <www.onevoice.ca>.

Osteoporosis Society of Canada, 33 Laird Drive, Toronto, ON M4G 3S9. Telephone: (416) 696-2663. Provides resources and a hotline for information about osteoporosis and menopause: in English, (800) 463-6842; in French, (800) 977-1778. Fax: (416) 696-2673. Website: <www.osteoporosis.ca>.

Pauktuutit Inuit Women's Association, 131 Bank Street, 3rd Floor, Ottawa, ON K1P 5N7. Telephone: (613) 238-3977. Fax: (613) 238-1787. E-mail: <pauktuut@comnet.ca>.

Psoriasis Society of Canada, P.O. Box 25015 Halifax, NS B3M 4H4. Telephone: (800) 656-4494. Fax: (902) 443-2073. Website: <www.psoriasissociety.org>.

Sex Information and Education Council of Canada (SIECCAN), 850 Coxwell Avenue, East York, ON M4C 5R1. Telephone: (416) 466-5304. Fax: (416) 778-0785. Publishes the *SIECCAN Journal* (see Newsletters and Periodicals). Website: <www.sieccan.org>.

Sleep/Wake Disorders Canada, 3089 Bathurst Street, Suite 304, Toronto ON M6A 2A4. Telephone: (800) 387-9253 or (416) 787-5374. Fax: (416) 787-4431.

South Asian Women's Centre, 1332 Bloor Street West, Toronto, ON M6H 1P2.

Thyroid Foundation of Canada, P.O. Box 1919, Main Station, Kingston, ON K7L 5J7. Telephone: (800) 267-8822 or (613) 544-8364. Fax: (613) 544-9731. Website: <www.thyroid.ca>.

Women's Health Interaction, 58 Arthur Street, Ottawa, ON K1R 7B9. Telephone: (613) 563-4801. Fax: (613) 594-4704. Resources related to reproductive health issues. Website: <www.web.net/~WHI>.

d. *A sampling of regional and local organizations. Some of these have been formed to deal with general issues of interest to women; some focus on health issues. (Listed from east to west.)*

Planned Parenthood Newfoundland/Labrador, 203 Merrymeeting Road, St. John's, NF A1C 2W6. Telephone: 1-877-NO-MYTHS or (709) 579-1009. Fax: (709) 726-2308. Website: <www.plannedparenthood.nf.ca>.

PEI Women's Network, P.O. Box 233, Charlottetown, PE C1A 7K4. Telephone: (902) 368-5040. Fax: (902) 368-5039.

East Prince Women's Information Centre, 4 Summer Street, Summerside, PE C1N 3H2. Telephone: (902) 436-9856. Fax: (902) 888-2344.

Second Story Women's Centre, 12 Dominion Street, Bridgewater, NS B4V 2W6. Telephone: (902) 543-1315. Fax: (902) 543-8653.

Planned Parenthood, P.O. Box 1598, Sydney, NS B1P 6R8. Telephone: (902) 539-5158. Fax: (902) 539-0290.

Centre des Femmes de Montréal, 3585 rue St-Urbain, Montreal, QC H2X 2N6. Telephone: (514) 842-4781. Fax: (514) 842-5613. Website: <www.cedep.net/~cfmwcm/>

Menopause Clinic, Sir. Mortimer B. Davis Jewish General Hospital, 3755 Côte Ste-Catherine Road, Montreal, QC H3T 1E2. Telephone: (514) 340-4933.

Lennoxville and District Women's Centre, P.O. Box 102, Lennoxville, QC J1M 1E3. Telephone (819) 564-6626. Fax: (819) 569-3199.

Menopausal Unit, Smythe Road Campus, Ottawa Hospital, 501 Smythe Road, Ottawa, ON K1H 8L6. Telephone: (613) 737-8556. Fax: (613) 737-8266.

Women's Place, 755 Somerset Street West, Dalhousie Community Centre, Ottawa, ON K1R 6R1. Telephone: (613) 231-5144. Fax: (613) 231-5270.

OSTOP Ottawa (Osteoporosis Self-Help Group), a self-help group for women interested in knowing more about osteoporosis, how to prevent it or how to deal with it. c/o Good Campanion Centre, 670 Albert Street, Ottawa, ON K1R 6L2. Telephone: (613) 236-0428. Fax: (613) 230-2095.

Sudbury Women's Centre, 324-E Elm Street West, Sudbury, ON P3C 1K4. Telephone: (705) 673-1916. Fax: (705) 673-7176.

Hastings and Prince Edward County Health Unit, Box 1080, 74A King Street, Picton, ON K0K 2T0. Telephone: (613) 476-7471.

Centre for Research in Women's Health, 790 Bay Street, 7th floor, Toronto, ON M5G 1N8. Telephone: (416) 351-3732. Fax: (416) 351-3746. Conducts and promotes research in women's health. Website: <www.utoronto.ca/crwh>.

City of Toronto Department of Public Health Resource Centre, 277 Victoria Street, 6th floor, Toronto, ON M5B 1W2. Telephone: (416) 392-7451.

College Street Women's Centre, 489 College Street, Suite 301, Toronto, ON M6G 1A5. Telephone: (416) 929-1816. Fax: (416) 929-3035.

East End Health Services, 343 Coxwell Avenue, Toronto, ON M4L 3B5. Telephone: (416) 778-5858.

Mature Women's Clinic, 655 Bay Street, Toronto, ON M5G 2K9. Telephone (416) 598-3523. Fax: (416) 598-4943.

Older Women's Network, 115 The Esplanade, Toronto ON M5E 1Y7. Provincial organization with four chapters in Ontario (Peterborough, Toronto, Hamilton, Waterloo). Membership is $25 for individuals, $50 for organizations, with a sliding scale.

Parkdale Community Health Centre, 1229 Queen Street West, Toronto, ON M6K 1L2. Telephone (416) 537-2455. Fax: (416) 537-5133.

Regional Women's Health Centre, 790 Bay Street, 8th floor, Toronto, ON M5G 1N9. Telephone: (416) 586-0211. Fax: (416) 351-5727. The centre has booklets about menopause in Spanish, Portuguese, Italian, Cantonese and Greek. Call or write for prices.

Smokefree Teaches Women to Quit Smoking, Broadview Avenue at the Danforth, Toronto, ON M4K 2P3. Addiction counselling and psychotherapy. Telephone: (416) 465-1323. Website: <www.smokefree.on.ca>.

Medical Reform Group, P.O. Box 366, Station J, Toronto, ON M4J 4Y8. A group of physicians committed to more equal access to health care and more emphasis on preventive aspects. Telephone: (416) 787-5246. Fax: (416) 782-9054. Website: <www.hwdn.org/ling/mrg>.

Toronto Endometriosis Association Support Group, P.O. Box 46026, College Park P.O., 44 Yonge Street, Toronto, ON M5B 2L8. Informal support group meetings held monthly. Open to the public. Meetings held at 790 Bay Street, 8th floor.

Toronto Women's Health Network, 1884 Davenport Road, Toronto, ON M6N 4Y2. Telephone: (416) 392-0898. Fax (416): 392-0645. Umbrella network of individuals and women's health organizations. Membership $18 for individuals. Publishes a monthly newsletter Website: <www.net/~twhn>.

Consumer Health Information Services, St. Joseph's Centre for Ambulatory Health Services, 2757 King Street East, Hamilton, ON L8G 5E4. Telephone: (905) 573-4810. Fax: (905) 573-4828. Website: <www.stjosham.on.ca>.

Planned Parenthood Society, 20 Hughson Street South, Suite 611, Hamilton, ON L8N 2A1. Telephone: (905) 528-3009.

Healthy Sexuality Program, Peel Health Department, 150 Central Park Drive, Suite 09, Brampton, ON L6T 2T9. Telephone: (905) 791-5905. Fax: (905) 789-1768. Website: <www.region.peel.on.ca>.

Guelph Community Health Centre, 176 Wyndham Street North, Suite #1, Guelph, ON N1H 8N9. Telephone: (519) 821-5363. Fax: (519) 821-5834.

Canadian Mental Health Association Community Support, 550 Hamilton Road, London, ON N5Z 1S4. Telephone: (888) 875-2944.

Women Today, 45 West Street, Goderich, ON N7A 2K5. Telephone: (519) 524-6767. Fax: (519) 524-1233.

Bruce Grey Owen Sound Sexual Health Unit, 920 First Avenue West, Owen Sound, ON K6V 5Y6. Telephone: (519) 376-9420.

Group Health Association, Women's Health Centre, 240 McNabb Street, Sault Ste. Marie, ON P6B 1Y5. Telephone: (705) 759-5552.

Women's Health Clinic, 419 Graham Avenue, 3rd floor, Winnipeg, MB R3C 0M3. Telephone: (204) 947-1517. Fax: (204) 943-3844. A community health centre run by and for women. Holds regular menopause clinics and information sessions and has an extensive resource centre. Website: <www.pangea.ca/~whc>.

Opaskwayak Cree Nation, Otineka Health Centre, Box 1000, The Pas, MB R9A 1L1. Telephone: (204) 627-7158.

Saskatoon Women's Network. Telephone (306) 249-4454.

Co-operative Health Centre, Resource Room, 110 8th Street East, Prince Albert, SK S6V 0V7. Telephone: (306) 763-6464. Fax: (306) 763-2101.

Grace Women's Health Centre, 1441 29th Street N.W., Calgary, AB T2N 4J8. Telephone: (403) 670-2270. Website: <www.crha.health.ab.ca>.

Menopause and You (Rae Garvey, R.N.) 4120–125th Street, Edmonton, AB T6J 2A3. Telephone: (780) 436-7164. Fax: (780) 939-8255.

Strathcona Family and Community Services, 21 Festival Way, Sherwood Park, AB T8A 5T8. Telephone: (780) 464-4044. Fax: (780) 449-1220.

Women's Resource and Drop-In Centre, 691A Fourth Avenue, Fernie, B.C. Telephone: (250) 423-4687. Fax: (250) 423-3633.

Health Action Network Society, 202–5262 Rumble Street, Burnaby, BC V5J 2B6. Telephone: (604) 435-0512. Fax: (604) 435-1561. Website: <www.hans.org>.

Women's Resource Centre, 7000 Minoru Boulevard, Suite 110, Richmond, BC V6Y 3Z5. Telephone: (604) 279-7060. Fax: (604) 279-7069. Website: <www.richmondwomenscentre.bc.ca>.

Vancouver Women's Health Collective, 175 East 15th Avenue, Suite #1, Vancouver, BC V5T 2P6. Telephone: (604) 736-4234. Fax: (604) 876-1282.

Women's Resource Centre, University of British Columbia, Vancouver, BC. Telephone: (604) 685-3934.

First Mature Women's Network Society, 411 Dunsmuir Street, 2nd floor, Vancouver, BC V6B 1X4. Telephone: (604) 681-3986. Monthly networking meetings, discussions, social health outreach program.

North Shore Women's Centre, 944 West 16th Street, North Vancouver, BC V7P 1R3. Telephone: (604) 989-6009.

Nelson District Women's Centre, 420 Mill Street, Nelson, BC V1L 4R9. Telephone: (250) 352-9916. Fax: (250) 352-7100.

East Kootenay Health Unit, Public Health Nursing Department, 1212 Second Street North, Cranbrook, BC V1C 4T6. Telephone: (250) 426-1314. Fax: (250) 426-1346.

Campbell River Women's Health Centre, 457–10th Avenue, Campbell River, BC V9W 4E4. Telephone: (250) 287-3044. Fax: (250) 287-3038.

Planned Parenthood Association, 285 Prideaux Street, Suite 204, Nanaimo, BC V9R 2N2. Telephone: (250) 753-9511.

Status of Women Action Group, P.O. Box 8989, Victoria, BC V8W 3S1. Telephone: (250) 383-7322. Fax: (250) 388-0100. Website: <www.pacificcoast.net/~swag>.

Victoria Faulkner Women's Centre, 503 Hanson Street, Whitehorse, YK Y1A 5M6. Telephone: (867) 667-2693. Fax: (867) 667-7004.

4. Publications which specialize or touch on issues of interest to the woman seeking to understand her body.

a. *Magazines about health. Some of these are better than others.*

Alive: Canadian Journal of Health and Nutrition. Published 12 times a year by Canadian Health Reform Products Ltd., Box 80055, Burnaby, BC V5H 3X1. $34 per year. Telephone: (800) 663-6513 or (604) 435-1919. Fax: (604) 435-4888.

FDA Consumer. Published 6 times a year by the U.S. Food and Drug Administration, Superintendent of Documents, P.O. Box 371954, Pittsburgh, PA 15250-7954. $16.88 (US) per year. Website: <www.fda.gov/fda>.

Health. Published 9 times a year by Times Publishing Ventures, P.O. Box 56863, Boulder, CO 80322-6863, U.S.A. $24 (CDN) per year. Telephone: (800) 274-2522. Website: <www.health.com>.

Herizons. Published quarterly at P.O. Box 128, Winnipeg, MB R3C 2G1. $23.99 per year. Telephone: (204) 774-6225.

Network/Le Réseau. Bilingual, quarterly publication on women's health published by the Canadian Women's Health Network, 419 Graham Avenue, Suite 203,Winnipeg, MB R3C 0M3. Membership is $10 for individuals, from $10-$20 for groups. Telephone: (888) 818-9172 or (204) 942-5500. Fax: (204) 989-2355. E-mail: <cwhn@cwhn.ca>.

Prevention: America's leading health magazine. Published monthly by Rodale Press, 33 East Minor Street, Emmaus, PA 18049, U.S.A. $15.94 (US) per year. Telephone: (800) 813-8070. Website: <www.prevention.com>.

b. *Newsletters and Periodicals.*

A Friend Indeed. A reliable, independent newsletter of information and support for women in menopause and midlife. Founded in 1984 by Janine O'Leary Cobb. Published six times a year by Initiatives for Women's Health, Inc., 419 Graham Avenue, Main Floor, Winnipeg, MB R3C 0M3. $34.20 per year in Manitoba; $32.10 elsewhere in Canada. Telephone: (204) 989-8028. Fax: (204) 989-8029. E-mail: afi@afriendindeed.ca. Website: <www.afriendindeed.ca>.

Alternatives: For the Health Conscious Individual. Published monthly by Mountain Home Publishing, P.O. Box 829, Ingram, TX 78025. $69(US) per year. Telephone: (800) 219-8591. Website: <www.drdavidwilliams.com>.

Alternative Therapies in Women's Health: Science-based information for clinicians. Published monthly by American Health Consultants, 3525 Piedmont Road, Building 6, Suite 400, Atlanta, GA 30305. $199 (US) per year plus GST. Telephone: (800) 688-2421 or (404) 262-7436. Fax: (800) 284-3291. Website: <www.ahcpub.com/ahc_root_html/products/ newsletters/atwh.html>.

Arthritis News. Published quarterly by The Arthritis Society and Rogers Media, Circulation Department, 777 Bay Street, 5th floor, Toronto, ON M5W 1A7. $14.95 a year. Telephone: (800) 217-0591. Fax: (416) 596-3498. Website: <www.arthritis.ca>.

Climacteric, the Journal of the International Menopause Society. Official publication of the International Menopause Society. Membership fee of $125 (US) per year includes a subscription. See listing under "International Organizations." Website: <www.imsociety.org>.

Consumer Reports on Health. Published monthly by Consumers Reports, Yonkers, N.Y. Order subscriptions from Box 56356, Boulder, CO 80322-6356. $24 (US) per year. Telephone: (800) 528-9648. Website:<www.consumer.org/resources/publications.htm>.

DES Action Voice. Published quarterly by DES Action USA for members. Memberships are on a sliding scale. Write to DES Action U.S.A., 610 16th Street, Suite 301, Oakland, CA 94612. Telephone: (510) 465-4011. Fax: (510) 465-4815. Website: <www.desaction.org>.

Endometriosis Association Newsletter. Published by Endometriosis Association, Inc. International Headquarters, 8585 North 76th Place, Milwaukee, WI 53223. Telephone: (414) 355-2200. Fax: (414) 355-6065. Website: <www.endometriosisassn.org>.

European Menopause Journal. Published quarterly by PMSI Bugamor BV, Rooseveltweg 15, 1314 SJ Almere, The Netherlands. $85 (US) per year.

Harvard Women's Health Watch. Published monthly by the Harvard Medical School Health Publication Group, P.O. Box 420068, Palm Coast, FL 32142-0068. $24 US. Telephone: (800) 829-5921. Website: <www.health.harvard.edu/newsletters>.

Health and Longevity. Published monthly by Dr. Willix's Health and Longevity, 14 West Mount Vernon Place, Baltimore, MD 21201. $85 (US) per year. Telephone: (410) 783-8960. Fax: (410) 783-8464.

Health Care for Women International. Published 8 times a year by Taylor and Francis Ltd., London, England. $41 (US) per year. Telephone: (215) 269-0400. Fax: (215) 269-0363. Website: <www.tandf.co.uk/journals/tf/07399332.html>.

HealthFacts. Published monthly by the Center for Medical Consumers, 130 McDougal Street, New York, NY 10012-5230. Telephone: (212) 674-7105. Fax:(212) 674-7100. $25 (US) per year. This is an excellent independent newsletter for those interested in medical issues. Website: <www.medicalconsumers.org>.

Health News: Your authoritative guide to current health issues. A consumer health letter published bimonthly by The Faculty of Medicine, University of Toronto, 92 College Street, Toronto, ON M5G 1L4. $24.95 a year. Telephone: (416) 217-0296. Fax: (416) 217-0378. Circulation/subscription enquiries: (416) 324-9191. Website: <www.strategicink.com/ uoft-healthnews/HNMain.html>.

Healthy Weight Journal. Excellent bimonthly publication on health and social concerns related to weight, including health risks of obesity. Decker Periodicals (Editorial): 402 South 14th Street, Hettinger, ND 58639. Telephone: (701) 567-2646. Fax: (701) 567-2602. Publishing and Circulation: 4 Hughson Street South, P.O. Box 620, LCD1, Hamilton, ON L8N 3K7. Telephone (800) 568-7821. Website: <www.health weightnetwork.com/hwj.htm>.

HerbalGram. Published quarterly by The American Botanical Council & Herb Research Foundation, Box 194345, Austin, TX 78714-4345. $50 (US) per year. Telephone: (512) 926-4900. Fax: (512) 926-2345. Scientific news about botanicals. Website: <www.herbalgram.org/>.

IPPF Medical Bulletin. Six issues yearly, published by the International Planned Parenthood Federation, Regent's College, Inner Circle, Regent's Park, London, England NW1 4NS. Summarizes medical and news reports related to Planned Parenthood's mandate. No charge. Telephone: 011 (44-171) 487-7900. Fax: 011 (44-171) 487-7950. Website: <www.ippf.org/pubs/medical/index.htm>.

Johns Hopkins Medical Letter: Health After 50. Published monthly by Subscription Department, P.O. Box 420148, Palm Coast, FL 32142. $36 (CDN) + GST per year. Telephone: (904) 446-4675. Website: <www.hopkinsafter50.com/>.

Journal of the American Medical Women's Association (JAMWA). Published bimonthly by the American Medical Women's Association, Journal Fulfillment, 801 N. Faircax Street, Suite 400, Alexandria, VA 22314. Free for members; $70 (US) for hard copy; $60 (US) online.

Journal of Women's Health. Published bimonthly by Mary Ann Liebert, 2 Madison Avenue, Larchmont, NY 10128. $213 (US) per year. Telephone: (914) 834-3100. Fax: (914) 834-3688. Website: <www.liebertpub.com>.

Maturitas: International Journal for the Study of the Climacteric. Official journal of the European Menopause and Andropause Society (EMAS). Published nine times a year by Elsevier Scientific Publishers, Journal Information Centre, 655 Avenue of the Americas, New York, NY 10010. Telephone: (212) 633-3750. Fax: (212) 633-3680. Subscription prices available from the publisher. Website: <www.elsevier.com/inca/publications/store/5/0/5/9/5/4/index.htt>.

Mayo Clinic Health Letter: Reliable information for a healthier life. Published monthly by Mayo Clinic Health Letter, P.O. Box 53886, Boulder, CO 80322-3886. $31 (US) a year. Telephone: (800) 666-3703. Website: <www.mayohealth.org>.

Melpomene: A journal for women's health research. Published three times a year by the Melpomene Institute (see U.S. organizations), 1010 University Avenue, St. Paul, MN 55104. $40 (US) membership fee includes a subscription. Focuses on the relationship between exercise and women's health. Telephone/Fax: (651) 642-1951. Website: <www.melpomene.org>.

Menopause: The Journal of the North American Menopause Society. Published bimonthly by Lippincott Williams and Williams, 352 West Camden Street, Baltimore, MD 21201-2436. $185 (US) per year. Telephone: (410) 528-4000. Website: <www.lwww.com>.

Menopause Management. Published bimonthly by Medquest Communications, Inc., 629 Euclid Avenue, Suite 1200, Cleveland, OH 44114. Complimentary with membership in NAMS (see "International Organizations"). Telephone (216) 522-9700. Fax: (216) 522-9707. Website: <www.menopause.org/projour/mmang.html>.

UNDERSTANDING MENOPAUSE

The Moisture Seekers Newsletter. Published nine times a year by the Sjögren's Syndrome Foundation Inc., 366 North Broadway, Suite PHW2, Jericho, NY 11753. Telephone: (800) 475-6473 or (516) 933-6365. Fax: (516) 933-6368. Website: <www.sjogrens.com>.

National Women's Health Network News. Published bimonthly at 514 Tenth Street N.W., Suite 400, Washington, D.C. 20004. Membership fee of $25 (US) includes the newsletter. Telephone: (202) 628-7814. Fax: (202) 347-1140. Website: <www.womenshealthnetwork.org>.

People's Medical Society. Published bimonthly by the People's Medical Society, Inc., 462 Walnut Street, Allentown, PA 18102. Membership fee is $24 (US) per year. Telephone (800) 624-8773 or (610) 770-1670. Fax: (610) 770-0607. Website: <www.peoplesmed.org>.

Public Citizen Health Letter. Published monthly by the Public Citizen Health Research Group, 1600 20th Street N.W., Washington, DC 20009. $18 (US) per year. Telephone: (202) 588-1000. Website: <www.citizen.org/hrg/>.

Radiance: The Magazine for Large Women. Upbeat and intelligent, Radiance includes personal stories, great fashions, and lots more to enhance self-esteem for women of all ages. P.O. Box 30246, Oakland, CA 94604. Telephone: (510) 482-0680. Fax: (510) 482-1576. Website: <www.radiancemagazine.com>.

SIECCAN: Canadian Journal of Human Sexuality. Published quarterly by The Sex Information and Education Council of Canada, 850 Coxwell Avenue, East York, ON M4C 5R1. Membership fee of $40 for individuals includes the journal. Telephone: (416) 466-5304. Fax: (416) 778-0985. Website: <www.sieccan.org>.

Society for Menstrual Cycle Research Newsletter. Published quarterly and sent to members. Annual fee is $35 (US). Membership secretary is Mary Anna Friederich, MD, 10559 North 104 Place, Scottsdale, AZ 85258. E-mail: <fmanna@uswest.net>. Website: <www.pop.psu.edu/smcr>.

Townsend Letter for Doctors and Patients: The Examiner of Medical Alternatives. Monthly publication on alternative therapies including an excellent update on women's health by Tori Hudson, N.D. Published by Townsend Letter Group, 911 Tyler Street, Port Townsend, WA 98368. Telephone: (360) 385-6021. Fax (360) 385-0699. Website: <www.tldp.com>.

Tufts University Diet and Nutrition Letter. Published monthly by Tufts University Diet and Nutrition, P.O. Box 57857, Boulder, CO 80322-7857. $25 (US) per year. Telephone: (800) 274-7581. Website: <www.healthletter.tufts.edu/>.

University of California at Berkeley Wellness Letter: The newsletter of nutrition, fitness, and stress management. Published monthly by Health Letter Associates, P.O. Box 420148, Palm Coast, FL 32142, U.S.A. $36 (CDN) + GST per year. Telephone: (904) 445-6414. Website: <www.berkeleywellness.com>.

Women's Global Network on Reproductive Rights. Published quarterly (in English and Spanish) by the organization of the same name, Vrolikstraat 453-D,

— 278 —

1092 TJ Amsterdam, The Netherlands. 70 Dutch guilders per year. Telephone: 011 (31-20) 620-9672. Fax: 011 (31-20) 622-2450. Website: <www.wgnrr.org>.

Women's Health. Published quarterly by Women's Health, London, England (see listing under "International Organizations"). Website: <www.womenshealthlondon.org.uk>.

Women's Health Journal. Published by the Latin American and Caribbean Women's Health Network, Coordinating Officer, Casilla 50610, Santiago 1, Chile. Telephone: 011 (56-2) 223-777. Fax: 011 (56-2) 223-1066. Website: <www.reddesalud.web.cl>.

Women's Health Issues. Published bimonthly by the Jacob's Institute of Women's Health, 409 Twelfth Street S.W., Washington, DC 20024-2182. $55 (US) for membership. Telephone: (202) 863-4990. Fax: (202) 488-4229. Website: <www.jiwh.prg/whi.htm>.

Women's Health Matters, 90 Eglinton Avenue East, Suite 403, Toronto, ON M4P 2Y3. $29.95 per year. Telephone: (800) 895-6434 or (416) 323-7322. Fax: (416) 813-4720. Website: <www.library.utoronto.ca/wch/wchmatters/intro.htm>.

GLOSSARY

adenomyosis
Condition where tissue from the endometrium becomes embedded in the muscle of the uterus itself.

adenosis
Abnormal development of a gland.

adhesions
Fibrous tissue that may form in any part of the body as a result of surgery, infection, or bleeding. Adhesions may scar organs together and, when removed surgically, may cause new adhesions to grow.

adrenal glands
Flattened body above each kidney that produces steroid hormones. The adrenals consist of a cortex and medulla. The cortex is responsible for many hormones, the medulla primarily for epinephrine (adrenaline).

agoraphobia
An irrational fear of being away from a known place. A common phobia among women, agoraphobia is diagnosed when panic attacks dictate a restricted area of activity for the phobic person. It can be effectively treated by behavior therapy.

air hunger
The temporary sensation of being starved of oxygen. Lasting only a few moments, this sensation is characteristic of pregnancy and menopause.

alendronate (Fosamax™)
Bisphosphonate approved for the prevention and treatment of osteoporosis.

alopecia
Absence or thinning of hair, a menopausal complaint common to women with a family tendency to male-pattern baldness. No recognized treatment exists, although estrogen (too much or too little) may have some influence.

alopecia areata
Patchy hair loss, usually reversible, in sharply defined areas, usually involving the scalp.

amenorrhea
Absence of menstruation for more than three cycles, usually

caused by fluctuating estrogen levels during breast feeding, heavy exercise, illness, stress, weight change, etc. Episodes of amenorrhea are characteristic of the perimenopause.

amines
Organic compounds containing nitrogen.

angina
Spasmodic, choking, or suffocating pain. Term used almost exclusively for chest pain (angina pectoris) usually due to interference with the supply of oxygen to the heart muscle and precipitated by excitement or effort.

aneurysm
A balloonlike swelling in the walls of a damaged artery.

anorexia nervosa
Condition based on fear of gaining weight, leading to extreme weight loss and amenorrhea. Anorexic patients are typically women in their late teens or early twenties. If not overcome, anorexia can lead to osteoporosis, heart disease, and, in some cases, to death as a result of self-starvation.

apnea
The cessation of breathing for a few seconds. Cause is unknown. Sleep apnea is believed responsible for some kinds of very loud snoring and may also be responsible for temporary episodes of "air hunger" during menopause.

areola
Area around the nipple of the breast. May be pink to dark brown.

arrhythmia
Any variation from a regular heartbeat, including tachycardia (too rapid) and bradycardia (too slow).

arteriosclerosis
Hardening of the arteries, a condition in which deposits form inside the arteries and affect blood flow from the heart.

artery/arteriole
Blood vessels that carry freshly oxygenated blood from the heart to all cells of the body.

aspirated
Drained of fluids by suction.

atheroma
Deposit of fats (or lipids) in the artery.

atherosclerosis
The formation of atheromas inside the walls of the arteries; part of the condition known as arteriosclerosis.

atrophic vaginitis
See dry vagina.

aura
A strange sensation that precedes the onset of a hot flash, a migraine headache, or an epileptic seizure. Auras may consist of visual disturbances, feelings of nausea, sudden changes in mood. The person having the aura learns that it is a signal of the onset of a flash, headache, etc.

basal skin cancer
Small, pink growths in the head or neck area. Over time, these change to a cluster of pimples and then to a deep, crusty sore.

benzodiazepines
Minor tranquilizers, also known as anxiolytics, often prescribed to menopausal women. The best known are lorazepam (Ativan), diazepam (Valium), and alprazolam (Xanax). These drugs may create psychological or physiological dependence and are depressants.

blepharoplasty
Medical term for eyelift.

bloat

The sudden distension of the waist or abdomen. Bloat may occur simultaneously with wind, or for no discernible reason. After a period of some discomfort (often two to three hours) it goes away. Common during premenstrual phase and menopause.

breakthrough bleeding

Bleeding or spotting between periods or after a long absence of periods (twelve months or more). Should be reported to a doctor.

BSE (breast self-examination)

A practice advocated by federal and provincial cancer societies to reduce the incidence of breast cancer. BSE should be practiced once a month and often locates lumps too small to be felt by an experienced physician.

bursitis

Inflammation of a fluid-filled sac or sacklike cavity (bursa). Bursae are situated in places like joints, such as the shoulder, where friction would otherwise occur.

calcitonin

A hormone produced by the thyroid that influences levels of calcium in the blood.

carcinoma in situ

A tumor where the tumor cells have not invaded the deepest membrane and are confined to the surface of the organ involved.

cerebral infarction

Death of brain tissue, often as the result of a stroke.

cerebral thrombosis

Blood clot in the brain.

cerebrovascular accident

See stroke.

cervicitis

Inflammation of the neck of the uterus.

cervix

The bottom third of the uterus that projects into the vagina. Viewed through the vagina, the cervix resembles a doughnut.

C.E.S.™ (ICN)

Generic form of conjugated estrogens (see Premarin).

cherry angioma

Round, bright red spot on the skin made up of blood vessels, often appearing for the first time during middle age.

cholesterol

Type of animal fat that is manufactured by the liver and circulated in the blood. Cholesterol is also eaten, primarily in the form of animal or dairy fats.

CHT (combined hormone therapy)

Also known as HRT. Usually understood to comprise ET with the addition of a progestational agent (synthetic progesterone – progestin or progestogen – or natural micronized progesterone) taken for a number of days in order to clear out possible excess cells from the uterus. Progestins may be taken monthly (the most common frequency) or, in particular cases, daily, quarterly, or semiannually. Women with no uterus may receive ET without a progestin.

climacteric

Generally used to refer to the middle years in both males and females, loosely the years from about forty to sixty. The word comes from a Greek term for ladder and signifies a new step every seven years. Historically, the climacteric was the years from forty-two to sixty-three, with the grand climacteric at the age of sixty-three.

Climacteron™ (Sabex)
Testosterone and estradiol injection used primarily to treat women after oophorectomy.

Climara™ (Berlex Canada)
Estradiol adhesive patch applied twice weekly to abdomen or buttock.

clitoris
A female organ, and the only human organ solely devoted to sexual pleasure.

clomiphene citrate
Generic drug widely known as the "fertility drug" and prescribed as Clomid (Arentis Pharma) or Serophene (Serono), an ovulatory agent that stimulates the release of gonadotropins (FSH and LH).

clonidine
Generic drug prescribed as Catapres or Dixarit (Boehringer Ingelheim). A drug used to control hypertension, which also acts to control hot flashes for some women.

collagen
A main supportive protein of skin, tendon, bone, cartilage, and connective tissue.

colporrhapy
An operation that tightens the supports under the neck of the bladder and removes the slack tissue of the vagina.

comedomastitis
See duct ectasia.

conization
The removal of a cone of tissue from the cervix for inspection and analysis.

corticosteroid
Any of the steroids produced by the adrenal cortex, or other natural or synthetic compounds with similar activity.

cystitis
Inflammation of the bladder, often producing a burning sensation when urinating.

D&C (dilatation and curettage)
A surgical procedure to clear out the uterus. The uterus is dilated and a long-handled spoon (the curette) is inserted to scrape out the interior surface. The procedure is essentially a blind one, since the surgeon cannot see the lining of the uterus.

danocrine
Generic term for the drug Cyclomen (Sterling-Winthrop), often prescribed for endometriosis, sometimes for premenstrual syndrome (PMS). It impedes ovulation and causes a pseudomenopause.

Delestrogen™ (Squibb)
Injectable estrogen (estradiol valerate) to treat the cessation of menstruation, irregular cycles, abnormal bleeding, menopausal symptoms, and to cause the endometrium to slough off.

dermabrasion
Planing of the skin done by mechanical means, e.g., sandpaper, wire brushes, etc.

diaphanography
Illuminating the breast with a very bright light to reveal the darker masses (potential tumors).

diastole
Force of the heart at rest.

digitalis
A genus of herbs (from the foxglove) used in the treatment of congestive heart failure.

dry vagina
A condition resulting from the thinning out of the vaginal walls and occurring either postmenopausally or as a result of surgical menopause (oophorectomy).

Also known as mature vagina.
Unacceptable terms are atrophic
or senile vagina.

duct ectasia
Dilation of the collecting (milk)
ducts of the breasts. Serious forms
of this are comedomastitis and
plasma cell mastitis.

duct hyperplasia
Abnormal growth of normal cells
of the lining of the milk ducts of
the breasts.

ductal carcinoma in situ (DCIS)
Common form of breast cancer
which, if left untreated, does not
develop into breast cancer in
80 percent of cases.

ductal papillomas
Benign growths (warts) in the
milk ducts of the breasts.

emphysema
A pathological accumulation of
air in tissues or organs.

endocrine
Bodily system comprising glands
that release hormones into the
bloodstream – i.e., pituitary,
thyroid, parathyroid, adrenals,
pineal body, gonads (ovaries or
testes), pancreas, and paraganglia.

endocrinologist
A doctor of internal medicine
who specializes in the diagnosis
and treatment of disorders of the
endocrine glands.

endometriosis
Abnormal occurrence of tissues
that more or less perfectly resemble the endometrium, in various
locations in the pelvic cavity.

endometrium
Tissue lining the uterus or womb.

epidemiologist
One who studies the relationships
of various factors determining the
frequency and distribution of diseases in the human community.

epidermis
The outermost, nonvascular layer
of skin.

ergotamine
Tartrate salt used for the relief
of migraine.

ERT (estrogen replacement therapy)
The term commonly (and
erroneously) used for estrogen
therapy. ERT is the correct term
only when referring to therapy
given to women who experience
either premature ovarian failure
or oophorectomy prior to normal
age at menopause.

Estrace™ (Roberts)
Estrogen (estradiol) tablets used
in ET, administered cyclically,
often coupled with progestogen/
androgen to prevent buildup of
endometrial tissue. Prescribed
for the relief of menopausal
symptoms.

Estracomb™ (Novartis)
Combination packet of Estraderm patches (see below) and
patches that combine estrogen
and a progestin.

Estraderm™ (Novartis)
Estradiol 17-beta in adhesive
patches that allow medication to
permeate the skin and move into
the circulation. Estraderm patches come in 25 mcg, 50 mcg, or
100 mcg and are usually worn for
three and a half days on the but-
tocks, abdomen, or thigh.

estradiol
A strong estrogen produced by
the ovaries. The major estrogen
in premenopausal women.

Estring™ (Pharmacia & Upjohn)
Vaginal ring designed to release
estrogen into the vagina over a
period of 12 weeks. For women
suffering from dry vagina.

estriol
The least powerful form of estrogen, a by-product of estrone.

Estrogel™ (Schering)
Estrogen gel applied to the abdomen for infusion through the skin.

estrogen
Hormone classified as "female sex hormone," although it is produced by both men and women. There are three major kinds of hormones: estradiol, estrone, and estriol.

estrone
A weak hormone produced partly by the ovaries and partly through the conversion, in body fat, of a precursor from the adrenal glands. Estrone is the main postmenopausal estrogen and the conversion process becomes more efficient with age.

ET (estrogen therapy)
Menopausal hormone therapy, the most common form being one tablet daily (or two patches weekly) for the first three and a half weeks of a month, with no estrogen from day 25 to day 30. There are many variations.

ethinyl estradiol
A common form of synthetic estrogen used in the contraceptive pill and, in much smaller quantities, in some forms of ET.

etidronate (Didrocal™)
Bisphosphonate approved for the prevention and treatment of osteoporosis.

fallopian tubes
Tubes with hairlike ends that pick up eggs erupting from the ovary and carry them down into the uterus.

fibrocystic
Characterized by an overgrowth of fibrous tissue and development of cystic spaces, especially in a gland.

fibroids
Colloquial clinical term for leiomyoma (benign tumors most often derived from smooth muscle) in or around the uterus.

fibromyalgia
The "sore-all-over" condition, also referred to as fibrositis. Symptoms include aching, pain, stiffness, sore spots that may continue for months or years. Diagnosis is often difficult and based on the presence of particular "tender spots." No cure, but can be relieved with proper treatment.

fibrosis
Firm mass in the breasts, difficult to distinguish from normal tissue. Usually benign.

fibrous dysplasia
See fibrosis.

follicle
Seedpod, or pouchlike covering surrounding the egg, or ovum, produced by the ovaries. When the follicle bursts, an egg is released to be picked up by the fallopian tubes.

FSH (follicle-stimulating hormone)
See gonadotropin. FSH is the agent that, during a normal menstrual cycle, induces follicles to develop and causes the lining of the uterus to thicken. When menopause is imminent, FSH levels in the blood increase enormously, and it is the presence of high levels of FSH that are considered confirmation of a menopausal state.

formication
A word used to describe the sensation of ants crawling on the skin, a common experience during menopause.

geriatrics
Department of medicine dealing with the problems of aging and diseases of the elderly.

gerontology
The scientific study of the problems of aging in all its aspects.

giant fibroadenoma
Rapidly growing rubbery tumor in the breasts.

gonadotropin
A substance that has a stimulating effect upon the ovaries, especially the hormone secreted by the anterior pituitary. Among such substances are follicle stimulating hormone (FSH) and luteinizing hormone (LH).

histamine
Amine that causes dilation of capillaries, constriction of the muscles in the lungs, increased gastric secretion.

homeopathy
Treatment of a disease by drugs, usually in minute doses, that in healthy persons would produce symptoms of the disease.

hormone
Substance produced by a gland and circulating through the bloodstream.

hot flash
The subjective sensation of heat, often through the chest and over the top of the head, but felt by some women to the ends of their fingertips and to the soles of their feet. There may be an accompanying rise in temperature. It is the most common menopausal complaint, but the cause is unknown.

hot flush
The evidence (red neck, face, enlarged veins, etc.) that often accompanies a hot flash. Not all hot flashes produce a flush. Not all flushes are felt as a flash. (In England, flush = flash.)

HRT (hormone replacement therapy)
The common term for combined hormone therapy, or CHT. Most synthetic hormones administered during menopause do not *replace* anything, since a decrease in estrogen and an absence of progesterone are normal for the woman undergoing natural menopause at an expected age.

hyperplasia
Abnormal increase in the number of normal cells in normal arrangement in an organ or tissue, which increases in volume.

hysterectomy
Surgical removal of the uterus. Complete hysterectomy involves removal of the uterus and cervix. Partial hysterectomy involves removal of the uterus only. Radical hysterectomy involves removal of the uterus, cervix, lymph nodes, and sometimes part of the vagina.

intraductal papillomas
Wartlike growths in the breasts that may produce a discharge from the nipple.

ischemic
Lacking oxygen.

labia
Lips (outer and inner) that cover female genitals.

laparoscopy
Procedure that may be diagnostic or operative. When used for diagnosis, it involves examination of the abdominal or pelvic cavity. A small incision is made in the

navel and carbon dioxide or nitrous oxide is pumped into the abdomen to give the doctor a better view of the pelvic organs. A laparoscope is then inserted, through which the doctor examines the pelvic organs. A second incision on the pubic line may be required for operative laparoscopy.

laparotomy
Incision through the abdominal wall.

LH (luteinizing hormone)
A gonadotropin, LH is responsible for inducing one follicle to ripen and burst.

lipectomy
Medical term for fat suction. Also lipolysis.

lipoma
A benign fatty tumor usually composed of mature fat cells.

lipoprotein
A combination of a lipid and a protein, having the general properties of proteins but categorized as high density, low density or very low density, etc. (HDLs, LDLs, VLDLs)

lithotomy position
Term used to describe position of woman during standard gynecological examination (i.e., knees spread, feet up on stirrups). This position is also used for certain types of hysterectomies, particularly for prolapsed uterus, and may involve tipping of the operating table so that the surgeon has a better view of the operating field. The result is often severe postoperative backache for the patient.

malignant melanoma
Form of cancer resulting from overexposure to the sun which begins as a raised, bumpy dark-ened area of skin. Its shape and color may change, and it may be itchy or sore.

mastitis
Inflammation of the breast.

menopause
Medical definition: the cessation of menstruation. Nonmedical definition: the years surrounding the cessation of menstruation.

Miacalcin™ (Novartis)
Calcitonin in a nasal spray, approved for prevention of spinal osteoporosis.

mitral valve
The valve between the left atrium and the left ventricle of the heart.

naturopathy
A drugless system of healing by the use of physical methods.

necrosis
Hard lump consisting of dead cells, often resulting from a blow.

Norlutate™ (Parke-Davis)
Androgenic form of progestin used in combination with ET to form CHT.

Oesclim™ (Fournier)
Self-adhesive estrogen patch.

Oestrilin™ (Desbergers)
Vaginal cones or vaginal cream used to treat dry vagina.

Ogen™ (Pharmacia & Upjohn)
Plant-based estropipate tablet used in ET.

oophorectomy (or ovariectomy)
Excision of one or both ovaries (both is a bilateral oophorectomy).

osteoarthritis
Degenerative joint disease accompanied by pain and stiffness.

osteomalacia
Softening of the bones due to a Vitamin D deficiency.

osteopenia
Any condition involving reduced bone mass.

osteoporosis
A condition of porous bone that may increase the risk of fracture.

palpitations
Disagreeable awareness of the heart beating.

pamidronate (Aredia™)
Bisphosphonate approved for treatment of Paget's Disease of the bone.

perimenopause
Period of time surrounding menopause when menstruation is irregular.

petrolatum
A purified mixture of hydrocarbons obtained from petroleum used as an ointment base or soothing application to the skin (e.g., Vaseline).

phlebitis
Inflammation of a vein.

placebo
Inactive substance given to substitute for active drug therapy. When a person believes that the pill (or treatment) will help, it helps in twenty to thirty percent of cases. Placebos are routinely used to test new medications: neither the individual nor the nurse or doctor giving the treatment knows whether it is a placebo or the real thing.

plasma cell mastitis
See duct ectasia.

postmenopause
Period of time when menstruation has definitely ceased. Postmenopause is usually understood to begin when a woman has not had a menstrual period for twelve months.

Premarin™ (Wyeth-Ayerst)
Tablet or vaginal cream containing conjugated equine estrogens used in ET.

premenopause
Period of time when some menopausal signs are present but before menstrual periods become irregular.

premenstrual syndrome (PMS)
A wide range of physical and emotional symptoms that precede (usually by seven to ten days) the menstrual period.

Premplus™ (Wyeth-Ayerst)
Combination tablets of conjugated equine estrogens and medroxyprogesterone acetate (see Provera).

prodrome
See aura.

progesterone
Hormone produced by the corpus luteum (yellow body) that is left after a follicle bursts from the ovary. This hormone paves the way for menstruation.

progestin or progestogen
Synthetic forms of progesterone. Generic names are medroxyprogesterone acetate, megestrol acetate, norethindrone, or norethisterone.

Prometrium™ (Schering)
Natural progesterone suspended in peanut oil, capsulated, used in CHT or to alleviate hot flashes for women who cannot take ET.

prostate
A gland surrounding the neck of the bladder and urethra in the male; it contributes a secretion to the semen.

Provera™ (Pharmacia and Upjohn)
Medroxyprogesterone tablets used in CHT or to prevent osteoporosis.

reserpine
An alkaloid used as an antihypertensive and tranquilizer.

rhytidectomy
Medical term for a facelift.

rickets
A condition caused by Vitamin D deficiency. Bones do not harden normally but are bent and distorted and have enlarged nodes at the ends and sides.

risedronate (Actonel™)
Bisphosphonate approved for treatment of Paget's Disease of the bone.

RNI (recommended nutrient intake)
Standards governing good nutrition developed by Health Canada.

senile lentigos
Liver spots caused by melanin (the dark pigment of the skin) deposits.

SERMs (selective estrogen receptor modulators)
Estrogens designed to confer the benefits of estrogen supplementation without the drawbacks. Some are more successful than others.

spironolactone
Generic name for an aldosterone (steroid hormone) inhibitor used as a diuretic. One trade name is Aldactone™ (Searle).

squamous cell cancer
Form of cancer that starts as a small, red, hard pimple and then becomes a hard, crusted sore that refuses to heal.

stilbestrol
Synthetic nonsteroidal estrogen, trade name Honvol™ (Horner) or Stilboestrol™ (Glaxo). Effects are similar to those of natural estrogens. Once used to prevent miscarriage, to dry up breast milk, and as a morning-after pill. Its legal use is now limited to the treatment of breast and prostate cancer.

stroke
A condition with sudden onset due to acute vascular lesions of the brain (hemorrhage, embolism, thrombosis, rupturing aneurysm), which may be marked by partial or total paralysis of one side of the body, vertigo, numbness, partial or total loss of speech, often followed by permanent neurologic damage. Medical terms are CVA (cerebro-vascular accident) or, in its milder form, TIA (transient ischemic accident).

suction curettage
Another term for fat suction, liposuction, or lipolysis.

systole
Force of the heart while pumping.

temporomandibular joint syndrome
(TMJ) Faulty articulation of the hinged joint of the jaw; a condition that may cause, in addition to headache, dizziness or ringing in the ears.

testosterone
A hormone secreted by the testes, which functions in the induction and maintenance of male secondary sex characters. A pharmaceutical compound is produced synthetically from cholesterol or isolated from bull testes.

thermography
Diagnostic technique that measures temperature differences between normal and abnormal (warmer) tissues. Useful, but by itself not accurate enough for diagnosing breast cancer.

thromboembolism
Obstruction of a blood vessel with thrombotic material carried by the blood from the site of origin to plug another vessel.

touch impairment
Sensitivity to being touched that makes one shrink from, or impedes, responses to touch. Nearly always temporary. Treatable with ET.

transillumination
See diaphanography.

tretinoin
Vitamin A acid cream used to modify wrinkles.

tubal ligation
Surgical technique of sterilization. The fallopian tubes are cut and bound, or plugged. Rarely reversible.

ultrasound
Technique that sends sound waves into the body that are reflected back onto a screen for display (also referred to as sonography).

uterus
A muscular organ, pear sized and shaped, part of the same structure as the cervix. Also known as the womb. The lining of the uterus is the endometrium. As well as holding the developing fetus, the uterus produces a substance called prostacyclin, which may influence the capacity for sexual response.

vasodilator
Causing dilation of blood vessels.

vasomotor
Referring to the veins and muscles. Hot flashes are vasomotor disturbances.

Viagra™ (Pfizer)
Product prescribed to stimulate sexual desire and enable erection.

withdrawal bleed
An artificial menstrual period, induced by CHT, assumed to eliminate the buildup of precancerous cells in the uterus.

INDEX

Since it began in 1984, many thousands of women have subscribed to **A FRIEND INDEED**, a newsletter for menopausal women published six times a year.

A FRIEND INDEED offers the latest news, views, research, and other items of interest to women who are approaching or experiencing menopause. Each issue also contains letters from readers, who share their personal experiences and remedies for menopausal complaints. In this way, **A FRIEND INDEED** not only informs but also provides a forum for women to share their feelings and experiences. It is a regular and dependable support to any woman in the prime of life.

Each issue of the newsletter consists of eight letter-sized pages, three-hole punched for handy filing in a three-ring binder.

A FRIEND INDEED can be reached at
<www.afriendindeed.ca>;
e-mail <afi@afriendindeed.ca>.

A one-year subscription can be ordered by
sending $32.10 (GST included) or
$34.20 from Manitoba (GST & PST included) to

A FRIEND INDEED
Main floor, 419 Graham Avenue
Winnipeg, MB R3C 0M3

(You can also pay by
Visa or Mastercard by calling
204-989-8028)